Praise for **Embrace Aging**

"Dr. Guerrasio's compassion for seniors shines throughout this book. With gentle humor and real-life examples, she convincingly conveys how everyone can live out our fullest lives healthfully and safely." **—Jane S. Kim**, MD, Geriatric Medicine Associates

"At last—a reasonable and common-sense approach to an elder patient's 'owner's manual.' Dr. Guerrasio's book provides helpful information on managing so many diverse medical and life issues. What I love about the book is the way she empowers her patients to take charge of their own heath care. I highly recommend this book for all of us to age well, with grace and vigor." **—Dr. C.**, author of *Possibilities with Parkinson's: A Fresh Look*

"This book helps you find your aging superpowers! Dr. Guerrasio uses patient stories, straightforward advice, and laughs to help you live your best life. I want her in my corner as I age!" **—Judy Zerzan-Thul**, MD, MPH, clinical associate professor, medicine, University of Washington, 2008–2009 Health and Aging Policy Fellow, and chief medical officer, Washington State Health Care Authority

"Dr. Guerrasio is an incredibly interesting and entertaining writer. She tells a story that you cannot wait to keep reading. I think this book might be the secret ingredient we all need as we contemplate aging. After reading *Embrace Aging*, I feel more confident about what my future holds." **—Natalie B.**, 52

"Dr. Guerrasio's book has challenged and changed me. Even though I am in the midst of my 87th year, I no longer consider myself aged or elderly, but aging. I am a work in progress. I loved Dr. Guerrasio's warmth, vast medical knowledge, and gentle humor, so present in the book. The way she engages the most difficult, complex, and uncomfortable subjects is remarkable. *Embrace Aging* is a resource for anyone, regardless of their age, wishing to move forward confident and well-informed as they address their ongoing journey." **—Jim B.**, 87

"*Embrace Aging* is so incredibly well written and easy to understand. Dr. Guerrasio is a brilliant doctor. Thank you for sharing this information." **—Barb F.**, 74

Embrace Aging

Conquer Your Fears and Enjoy Added Years

Jeannette Guerrasio, MD

Rowman & Littlefield
Lanham • Boulder • New York • London

Published by Rowman & Littlefield
An imprint of The Rowman & Littlefield Publishing Group, Inc.
4501 Forbes Boulevard, Suite 200, Lanham, Maryland 20706
www.rowman.com

86-90 Paul Street, London EC2A 4NE, United Kingdom

British Library Cataloguing in Publication Information Available

Library of Congress Cataloging-in-Publication Data

Names: Guerrasio, Jeannette, 1977- author. | Guerrasio, Jeannette, editor.
Title: Embrace aging : conquer your fears and enjoy added years / Jeannette Guerrasio, MD.
Description: Lanham : Rowman & Littlefield, [2022] | Includes bibliographical references and index.
Identifiers: LCCN 2021056590 (print) | LCCN 2021056591 (ebook) | ISBN 9781538164228 (cloth) | ISBN 9781538164211 (epub)
Subjects: LCSH: Older people. | Well-being—Age factors. | Self-help techniques.
Classification: LCC HQ1061 .G854 2022 (print) | LCC HQ1061 (ebook) | DDC 305.26—dc23/eng/20211117
LC record available at https://lccn.loc.gov/2021056590
LC ebook record available at https://lccn.loc.gov/2021056591

∞™ The paper used in this publication meets the minimum requirements of American National Standard for Information Sciences—Permanence of Paper for Printed Library Materials, ANSI/NISO Z39.48-1992.

To Bill and Jock, never forgotten.

Disclaimer

This book is meant to serve as a general guide for a better understanding of common health problems. It is not individualized to your specific health situation. The goal is to serve as education that you can use when interacting with your healthcare providers. Always seek the advice of your physician or other qualified healthcare providers with any questions you may have regarding a medical condition, including advice, diagnosis, and treatment. Never disregard professional medical advice or delay in seeking it because of something you have read in this book.

Product names are provided for information and not an endorsement.

All patient stories are amalgams of real patients that I have seen in the past. All identifying information has been removed to protect patient privacy.

CONTENTS

ACKNOWLEDGMENTS

My sincerest thank you to my biggest fan, who has supported my personal and professional development in innumerable ways. Lara Juliusson gets full credit for drawing and digitizing all of the illustrations, which I then labelled. She also managed our small zoo of dogs and cat in the evenings so that I could have less interrupted time to complete this writing project. Every moment with you is a treasure, and I want to thank you for sharing our time for the benefit of others.

I am deeply grateful to all of my patients who I truly enjoy and from whom I have learned so much. You have been so generous in your sharing over the years. Special thank you to my friends: David Mellman, MD, who is the best colleague to collaborate with and human being to spend every day with; photographer Sarah Pollock who not only took my headshot while standing precariously on a windowsill but for also helping me manage my practice of patients at the same time; poet and editor Max Regan, MFA, who sparked my interest in writing and who has been a great guide; Ethan Cumbler, MD, who helped foster my love of geriatrics and has a solution to every problem; Nancy Novosad Bader for reviewing all of my writing and engaging me in the most stimulating conversations; and Barbara Stanton for reviewing my very rough first draft and for your ever thoughtful comments that have made this book so much better. Of course, thank you to my mom and dad who also helped review the first draft and, as the proud and supportive parents that they are, commented "Everyone should get a copy!" Thank you to them for my sense of humor, my love of people and medicine. Thank you to nephew and niece, Jared and Hailey, and cousin Janice (one of my many amazing cousins) for letting me use some of their personal stories.

With much gratitude, I wish to thank my literary agent, Joan Parker from Parker Literary Agency, LLC, who has worked tirelessly to guide me through the publication process (yet again!) and to find the perfect publisher to represent this work. It's been a pleasure working with Suzanne Staszak-Silva and the entire crew at Rowman & Littlefield, and I am honored to be working with such a great publishing company.

INTRODUCTION
Welcome to Aging

It's Never Too Late

No matter how old you are when you get your hands on this book, it is never too early or too late to adjust the trajectory of your aging process. As long as you are still here on Earth, there is time to take agency of your life, your body, and your mind. How we age is up to us!

I met Mae in the hospital. She was ninety-three years old. A stumble over her cat led to a fall, as well as a laceration on her head, that landed her in the hospital. When she fell, she was unable to recover quickly, and she struck her head on a table. The cut bled quite a bit due to her blood-thinning medications. She lived alone and knew she should call for an ambulance to take her to the hospital. In the emergency department, they cleaned up her wound, stapled it closed, checked a CT scan of her head, and asked her to stay the night for observation since she had hit her head. The next morning, I saw her working with physical therapy in the hall before she went home.

Mae was wearing the hospital-issued lime-green hospital gown, tied tightly in the back. Of her own, she wore her brown silk cap, white socks, and fuchsia-pink Saucony sneakers.

As I complimented her sneakers, she politely corrected me and said, "These are my marathon shoes."

"What?!? You have marathon shoes!" I exclaimed.

"Well, I used to run marathons until I was eighty-eight. Now I walk, and since no one can wait for me to finish, I just walk half-marathons."

"Good for you!" I replied with a proud smile on my face.

I felt truly proud for this woman who I barely knew. Her story is one of hope and empowerment. She was ninety-three, yet she still lived at home, took care of herself and her home, moved independently, and was doing the things she wanted to do. She was full of life. She demonstrated a recurrent message in my practice: How we age is up to us!

Power of Aging

We live in a culture in the United States that has, what I believe, a misguided devaluation of elders and an overemphasis on the magic of youth. Just picture the cities of Europe, with street after street lined with beautiful, resilient, historic, and powerful architectural buildings from 400 to 500 years ago. As we age, we, too, become more resilient, gain wisdom through history, and find our power. With age, people become clearer in their priorities and values, learn to show more empathy and support to those around them, and become more beautiful to their families and loved ones.

Taboo Subjects

Some people find it difficult to talk or even read about topics associated with aging. They struggle with embarrassment and shame in acknowledging that their lives and bodies are changing in ways they hadn't expected. This is also a feature of the culture in which we live, and I respect that sense of discomfort. In this book, I address topics that some may find uncomfortable. It was very important for me to acknowledge all of the concerns that I hear every day from my patients, knowing that other people may have the same questions and curiosities but are more hesitant to ask. My goal is to address all the challenges of aging and to provide strategies so that you can live your best life.

It is so important for you to find a doctor that you can talk to about anything and everything, including topics that feel taboo to you. If you have a doctor that you don't feel comfortable talking to about everything, then something important might get missed. Please find another doctor that respects you, truly values the gifts that you and other aging people bring to our communities, and is willing to listen, validate, and address your concerns.

What Age Is Considered Old?

Our communities are full of empowering, optimistic, and hopeful stories about people succeeding through their senior years. The term "senior citizen" traditionally referred to those greater than sixty-five years of age. But for many, sixty-five still feels young, so the phrase "old-old years" was invented to refer to those over eighty-five. I feel so lucky to be able to work in my current practice that affords me time to do both office visits with ample time to see patients and also to do house calls whenever requested. We have so many "old-old" patients who are living independently at home alone or with their similarly aged spouses. While they may not feel comfortable driving in the city anymore to come to the doctor's office, I want to promote and support their ability to live independently. They still have amazingly full lives, and they hold the secrets to conquering aging, and this book is filled with their stories and shared wisdom.

I walked into Charlie's house, and he was sitting in his usual seat on one end of his two-person sofa. There was a pile of new, partially read newspapers on the seat cushion to his right. His walker was in front of his legs, serving as an end table for his coffee mug and pen. I set my quintessential black leather doctor bag down and sat across from him on another sofa. There was just enough room for my bottom on one end and his visiting son Charles Junior to sit on the other end of this second sofa. Between us was a stack of old newspapers, which I presumed were from earlier in the week.

Charlie was wearing his usual khaki pants over his long johns, with suspenders strapped over his flannel button-down shirt with a white T-shirt showing underneath. He preferred his brown sheepswool-lined slippers for his arthritic ankles and feet. There wasn't much to keep the top of his head warm, except for a horseshoe ring of fine hair that ran on the back of his head from ear to ear. He had fine white hair that, despite being two inches long, always stood out from his head at the direction of its choosing. His skin was a pale white, and his eyes were dark blue, but today, the sparkle was gone, and the usual smile was replaced with a serious mask of concern.

I had planned to greet him with a big, "Happy Birthday!" but read the room quickly, and instead, I asked, "How are you feeling?"

He reported stoically, attempting to hide the fear in his voice, "I had a dream last night, that I was driving into a big billboard, and it said ninety-five!"

"What scares you about being ninety-five?" I asked.

"Well, not dying. I tried that five years ago when my kidneys started to fail, and I'm still here. It's just that, well . . . I just never felt *old* before."

I never stop learning from my patients. Just the night before, I had yet another menopausal hot flash. The kind that starts with the sensation of a combustion engine being started in the depths of your soul, leaving your pajamas soaked in a humid sweat followed by a shivering wet and cold. Admittedly, I felt a bit embarrassed that a hot flash made me feel like I was getting old.

I reflected back to him with genuine curiosity, "You never felt old before ninety-five?"

"You and your partner have been great doctors and teachers. I've always known what to expect with my body through the years and have always been able to prepare and plan. I guess now I just don't know what comes next."

"There is always another chapter. You are still here, and at ninety-five, there is still time to take some agency over life's aging process. I want to hear more of your concerns so I can advise you on the next steps." And so, we did.

On a subsequent home visit, I watched the joy in his eyes as he spoke so complimentary of his adult granddaughter, who was in the room with us. She was a pure delight as she then discussed her future plans of joining the AmeriCorps after college before starting professional school. They clearly had an amazing connection. He expressed such gratitude that he had lived long enough to see her into adulthood. Last month, he turned ninety-six.

Learn as Much as You Can

My patients have given of themselves so selflessly over the years. They have filled my mind with their curious questions about their bodies, their health, their afflicted diseases, and their future goals and dreams. They have encouraged me to continuously read on new innovations in medical diagnoses and treatment and to expand my understanding of medicine well beyond that of prescribing pills. They have helped me perfect the art of medicine and encouraged me to grow my skills as a teacher.

I've always believed that education is power, as do my patients. Charlie never felt old because he felt prepared. He knew how his body was supposed to change over time. He felt like he was on the trajectory that he was meant to be on. He felt empowered by his age. I want to get rid of the notion that aging should be reversed or that only young people have a fulfilling, enjoyable life. Every time I see Charlie, he tells me something he did that made him happy.

Personal Capacity and Hope

I'm writing this book during the COVID-19 pandemic. When the pandemic hit, I worried about my senior patients who would be most vulnerable to social isolation, especially those who lived alone. To stay connected, I started writing weekly newsletters to the patients in our practice that addressed ways to support one's mental health, provided updates about the virus, and summarized one new health topic per week. It also included a section that responded to questions that patients had sent to the practice via email. It was a way for me to build a community and keep people feeling united. Now patients submit photos, quotes, poems, and book suggestions that get added to the newsletter.

It was the feedback that I received from the newsletters that led to this book. But COVID-19 has done more than encourage me to write a book that would help others age better; it has taught me about a person's capacity to help themselves and how to maintain hope for the duration. If I want to better protect myself from patients with COVID-19, I can wear a mask and a face shield or glasses. I can read and learn everything there is to learn about the virus. I can follow the recommendations of Dr. Anthony Fauci. I can limit my in-person social interactions. I can go to the grocery store when it is less crowded. I can postpone my vacation for a year or two. I have control over what happens to my life. Aging is no different. Every day, I live with hope as information about the new vaccines and treatments emerge. Just because we don't have ideal treatments today doesn't mean there won't be one tomorrow. The same is true for some of our most challenging obstacles of aging. Research on dementia, for example, is continuous. Just because my grandfather had Alzheimer's dementia doesn't mean that if I were to get it, there won't be better treatments or even a cure in the future.

The aging process is normal, but we still can influence the way we age and have hope for the future. This book is designed to help people understand what is happening to their bodies. Everyone reads books when they are pregnant about how their body is changing. It is just as important to understand how your body is changing now, too. Remember the stories of Mae and Charlie. Your body can change and will change, and you can still have a wonderfully fulfilling life as you age. The more you know, the more you can do and the better prepared you will be. You are more empowered to affect the future than you think you are.

I made the comment about menopause earlier. Some women start worrying about aging as they go through menopause, losing their libido and fertility. Men may start to worry about aging as their plumbing doesn't work as well, with multiple nightly trips to the bathroom and less-reliable erections. The truth is aging starts around age thirty for every organ of the body. By the time you realize that you are aging, you have already been conquering it for twenty years! My goal is to help you understand it better so that you can be an active participant filled with hope rather than a passive observer filled with worry. Living your best life isn't just about a pill your doctor can give you; it is about the options we have and the choices we make. Yes, aging can be scary and fraught with unexpected challenges, which I prefer to call adventures. We will discuss that too. I hope to present you with all the medical advice you need to make better choices for yourself so that your aging life is happy, independent, fulfilling, and satisfying.

CHAPTER ONE

OSTEOARTHRITIS: I'M FINE BUT EVERYTHING HURTS

Living with Osteoarthritis

I have dozens of patients that are lucky enough to have lived ninety-five years without any serious health problems. They take no medications, except an occasional acetaminophen (Tylenol). They have never had surgery or been hospitalized, yet they all have the same complaint—"Everything hurts." Years of wear and tear on their joints have led to osteoarthritis. The soft cartilage cushions that once existed between the bones in their joints have been slowly filed away with every bend and release.

One of my eighty-three-year-old patients, who is still an active skier, has a great saying: "If you rest, you rust!" The activity that keeps her vital organs healthy, her brain functioning in tip-top shape, and has allowed her to maintain an active life, unfortunately, has also resulted in arthritis. Her goal and my goal for her is to find a way to overcome this challenge so that she can continue to participate in her activities without pain limiting her. I was confident in our success when she passed me on the ski slopes this winter.

A Universal Challenge

If you are over fifty, chances are you have some nagging arthritis somewhere in your body that flares up from time to time. Do your knees remind you that you went hiking yesterday? Does your lower back remember the heavy box you carried this morning? Are your thumb joints as angry with the Pickleball racket as you are? The truth is you don't have to be old to experience arthritic pains. Osteoarthritis begins developing at the age of thirty. How you have used your bony skeleton over the years will determine when you start to feel that early morning achy joint stiffness, which joints will be involved and how quickly it will progress. If you were a linebacker on a football team or a catcher for your softball team, you would likely develop arthritis in your knees before your friend who joined the band instead. Genetics also plays a large role in how your arthritis develops. Take a look at your hands. Do they look like mom's hands or dad's? If they look like mom's and she had very little arthritis, then you are lucky. If they look like mom's and she had terrible arthritis, let's talk about being prepared.

Osteoarthritis Is Not Inflammatory

Before we move on, I want to clarify that osteoarthritis is very different from other types of inflammatory arthritides, like rheumatoid arthritis, psoriatic arthritis, or gouty arthritis. In these types of arthritides, one's own immune system attacks their joints or crystals form in the joints as with gout, causing an inflammatory reaction that erodes the joint. I like to think of osteoarthritis as more of a mechanical problem. Eventually, the tire treads on your car, the brake pads on your bike, and/or the soles of your shoes just wear out.

Symptoms and Stages of Osteoarthritis

Osteoarthritis causes joint pain, stiffness, and restriction in movement in one or more joints. It is usually not symmetric but can become symmetric over time. Knees, hips, hands and fingers, neck (cervical spine), and lower back (lumbar spine) are most frequently affected and in that order. However, if you were a competitive swimmer, you might be more likely to get shoulder arthritis. The symptoms can seem somewhat paradoxical. The pain and stiffness can be worse in the morning if you haven't been moving much all night until you get up and get moving. This limitation should improve within thirty minutes. At the same time, the more you use a joint, the more it tends to hurt. So, it also tends to hurt in the late day, if you have been using the joint repetitively. Then the discomfort is relieved by rest. For example, Carol's hands are stiff for fifteen minutes in the morning until she gets them moving, and then by the end of the day, the achiness returns to her knuckles and wrists after crocheting her grandson's baby blanket. If she rests her hands while reading a book for a few hours, they will feel better again as long as she doesn't rest for too long.

Osteoarthritis has three stages:

Stage 1: The first stage is predictable, with sharp pain brought on by high-impact activities and very limited effect on day-to-day function. For example, your left knee hurts after a long run, but you can still climb the stairs to get into bed at night, shower the next morning, and head off to work.

Stage 2: Now the pain is more constant and affects your daily activities. The stiffness at times may seem unpredictable. For example, your knee hurts all the time, and you decide not to go to the store this afternoon because you will have to park far away from the entrance. You plan on going tomorrow morning because you can get in and out quicker . . . taking fewer steps.

Stage 3: By this stage, an individual has constant dull/aching pain with unpredictable, intense, exhausting pain that severely limits their function. By now, someone else is going to get your groceries for you, or you've resorted to using a scooter.

While there are three progressive stages to osteoarthritis, progression is highly variable, and it is possible to remain at one stage for indefinite periods of time. Osteoarthritis can lead to tenderness of the joints, limited motion of the joints, bony swelling most noticed on the fingers, and joint deformities. It then often leads to sequelae like weak and fatigued muscles, overcompensation injuries on healthier joints, and poor balance, all of which are treatable.

Diagnosing Osteoarthritis

Physical exams and X-rays are the best way to diagnose osteoarthritis. Your doctor will look for the following (see Figures 1.1 and 1.2):

- Effusions—an abnormal presence of fluid in the joint, which is felt for on physical examination
- Osteophytes—bony lumps, also referred to as bone spurs
- Joint space narrowing—when the cartilage is gone, the distance between bones on X-ray disappears
- Subchondral sclerosis—a hardening or thickening of the bone under where the cartilage should be
- Cysts—fluid-filled areas that are inside

MRIs are often not necessary as they are more frequently used to show soft-tissue structures like tendons, ligaments, and crescent-shaped cartilage (menisci) rather than bone. Ultrasound is another imaging modality that can be useful to see fluid in the joint that can occur with osteoarthritis and osteophytes but is very operator-dependent. You have to have a very skilled technician performing the test to get accurate results.

Devising a Treatment Plan for Osteoarthritis

When your doctor considers a treatment plan for you, they are considering many aspects of your health and life:

- Previous treatments you have tried
- Impact of the pain and any functional impairment on you and your life
- Your ability to participate with a treatment plan and any possible restrictions—financial, getting to appointments, other life obligations
- Recreational and occupational goals
- Mood
- Sleep disturbances
- Fall risk
- Other active and chronic medical diseases
- Expectations of treatment
- Risk factors that you can help change like body weight, the angle of your joints (joint alignment) through exercises, the use of insoles in your shoes (Orthotics) or support braces for the joints, and your ability to adopt injury prevention techniques

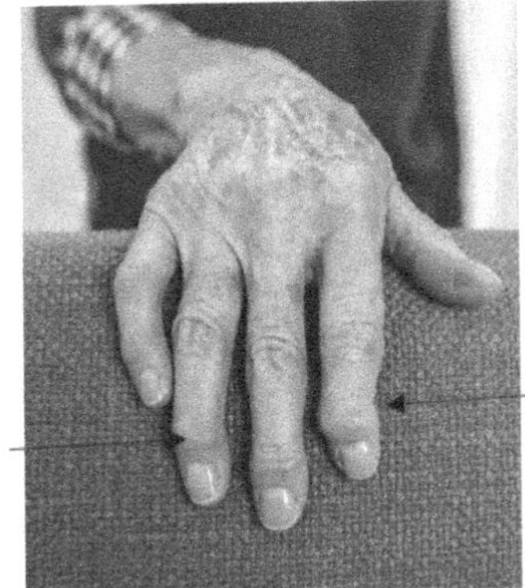

Figure 1.1. A 78-year-old hand with osteoarthritis. Courtesy of the author.

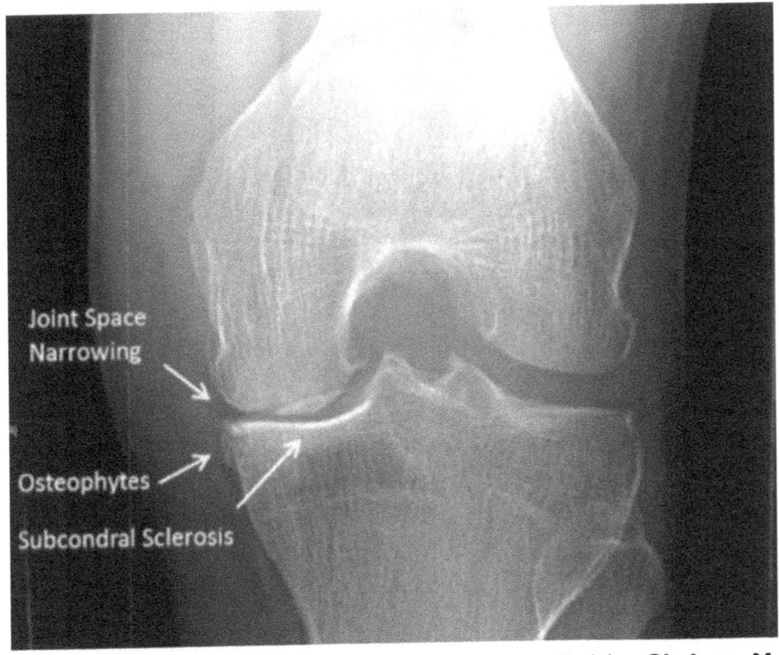

Figure 1.2. A 65-year-old knee with osteoarthritis. Oladapo M. Babatunde, Jonathan R. Danoff, David A. Patrick, Jonathan H. Lee, Jonathan K. Kazam, and William Macaulay. "The Combination of the Tunnel View and Weight-Bearing Anteroposterior Radiographs Improves the Detection of Knee Arthritis." ***Arthritis*** **(January 26, 2016): 1–8. https://doi.org/10.1155/2016/9786924**

Your doctor will then use this information to minimize your pain, optimize your ability to function while limiting the chance of injury, and help you achieve your goals. Each treatment in the doctor's black bag, so to speak, is of modest effect, so multiple treatments are required to see improvement. Please notice that I didn't say cure (at least not at this time). Many of the treatments are aimed at managing the effects rather than delaying the progression of osteoarthritis.

What You Can Do for Yourself

- Maintain a healthy body weight with a goal body mass index (BMI) of 22–27. Data suggests that people over sixty-five with a slightly higher BMI goal range have lower mortality than the BMI range of 19–25 recommended for younger adults. Your BMI can be calculated online or else the equation is:

  $$\text{BMI} = \text{your weight in kilograms} / (\text{your height in meters})^2$$

- Ice for twenty minutes to the painful joint several times per day, with heat to surrounding muscles if strained from osteoarthritis.
- Participate in physical therapy and continue to do your exercises between and after sessions have ended.
- Work with a trainer or physical therapist to correct postural and gait imbalances that create asymmetric wear and tear on your joints.
- Avoid repetitive activities, use tools to lessen strain on the joints or at least take breaks. For example, after typing at the computer for hours, do stretches to correct your hunched-over posture. Use a device to make opening jars easier so as not to put wear and tear on hand joints.
- If recommended by your doctor or physical therapist, wear braces, splints, and orthotics as appropriate, and other assistive devices.
- Try topical over-the-counter medications such as diclofenac gel (Voltaren®), CBD creams, and/or capsaicin. If you use

capsaicin, be sure to wash your hands before you touch your face. It contains pepper!

- Oral anti-inflammatory medications such as oral acetaminophen (Tylenol®), ibuprofen (Motrin®), naproxen (Aleve®), celecoxib (Celebrex®), and meloxicam (Mobic®) are great for arthritis; just ask your doctor before starting these medications and find out if it is safe for you to take them every day.
- Seek treatment for depression and sleep disorders, both of which are known to worsen pain.
- In terms of supplements, some use the following: Vitamin D, diacerein, avocado soybean unsaponifiables, and fish oil. Unfortunately, none of these have shown benefits in trials. Curcumin found in turmeric, Boswellia serrata, and glucosamine with chondroitin have shown some preliminary evidence of potential benefit, though the effects are modest. Several of my patients really like Joint Synergy, though I don't know that there is data on the efficacy of this product.
- Some people find acupuncture and transcutaneous nerve stimulation to be helpful; others do not. They are not dangerous and may be worth the try.

What Your Doctor Can Do

- Confirm the diagnosis and monitor its progress.
- Support your weight-loss goals and provide some accountability by having you report in regularly with your progress.
- Order physical therapy and suggest and prescribe assistive devices or orthotics.
- Ensure that it is safe for you to use over-the-counter medications and supplements.
- Help you find a therapist and/or prescribe duloxetine, which is an antidepressant that has been shown to help with pain.
- Give you steroid injections into the joint (intra-articular glucocorticoid injections), which provide short duration improvements from four weeks to a year. The long-term outcomes are variable.

- Provide injections into the joint with a chemical called hyaluronic acid. Hyaluronic acid is a clear, gooey substance that your body naturally makes. It helps retain water and keep body parts lubricated. The hope is that when placed in a joint, it will help lubricate moving parts and allow the joint to move with less pain. It is important to know that these injections are very expensive and lack clinical data to show significant benefits over placebo.
- Discuss and recommend surgical options, including joint replacements, which are available for many joints, including knees, hips, shoulders, ankles, and fingers. However, 9 to 20 percent of people have moderate to severe long-term pain after surgery. Higher rates of pain depend on how much pain is coming from the soft tissue (ligaments, tendons, muscles) around the joint prior to surgery, as well as any surgical complications. Arthroscopic surgery has shown no clinically significant benefits over non-surgical treatment or placebo. Therefore, it is not recommended.

Of note, a 10 percent loss of body weight (if overweight) and exercise results in a 50 percent decrease in pain after eighteen months for knee pain and likely hip pain, though hips specifically have not been studied. Exercise alone has a similar magnitude of effect as anti-inflammatory medications. Tai chi was studied and determined to be at least as effective as physical therapy for osteoarthritis.

When starting an exercise program or physical therapy, you must warm up and stretch five to ten minutes prior to beginning. Tendons, ligaments, and cartilage have less water in them as you age due to dehydration, which is explained in chapters 14 and 17, and because they are drier, they are more likely to tear. You too, runners! You have to stretch before you head out if you want to spare yourself from injury. (If you are not a runner, runners have a bad habit of just going for a run and end up with tight joints, especially in the hips and lots of soft-tissue injuries from not stretching.)

The Future of Osteoporosis

The next frontier is exploring cooled radiofrequency ablation of nerves to control osteoarthritis pain. The early results have been hopeful. New monoclonal antibodies like canakinumab are even being explored to help prevent the progression of osteoarthritis.

I don't want you to become sedentary so that you don't develop osteoarthritis. Remember that my wise patient pointed out that you just might rust, metaphorically speaking! I want you to be able to live life the way you want. You can do this by starting the lifestyle modifications mentioned in this chapter now, such as maintaining a normal weight, stretching and exercising, working to correct any body asymmetries, and avoiding repetitive motions that lead to injury. This will delay damage to your joints, reduce pain, and lessen the need for more aggressive therapies like joint replacements. If you opt not to treat your arthritis, it will lead to immobility and a decline in overall health and mental well-being, which is associated with a shorter life span. If you already have bad arthritis, it is not too late to start working on a plan to get your life back, one step at a time.

CHAPTER TWO

OSTEOPOROSIS: FALLING DOESN'T MEAN YOU HAVE TO BREAK!

Unexpected Breaks

I had the lovely opportunity to teach medicine in Melbourne, Australia, for a month. What made the trip even more memorable was that I invited my colleague Juan to join me as a co-teacher to share in the adventure. We decided to spend one extra week in Australia to go see the little blue penguins on Phillip Island and explore the Great Ocean Road. On our first free day, I stepped off the bus onto an uneven rain gutter and rolled my right ankle. After a few moments of silence, I joked to ease the other passengers, "Thank goodness I'm not old, otherwise that ankle sprain would have been a broken bone!"

I got up and told Juan he would have to drive the rest of the trip, on the opposite side of the road no less. I bought a cane at the gift store, and Juan helped me wrap my ankle. We proceeded to watch the most incredible migration of hundreds of twelve-inch penguins as they scurried from the water to their burrows, successfully avoiding predators from the sky. I eventually did get an X-ray, and with a chuckle, I reported the results to Juan: "I guess I am an old lady. Fractured times two."

Preventable? In so many ways.

CHAPTER TWO

What Is Osteoporosis?

One of my many goals is to help you understand osteoporosis and to help reduce your number of lifetime fractures. First, let's just review the anatomy of the bone. The bone is covered with a thin layer called the periosteum. Under the periosteum is compact bone. The center of the bone is filled with spongy bone with cross-links called trabeculae (see Figure 2.1).

As bones become thinner, the cross-links break down, and there are fewer and thinner trabeculae to stabilize the strength of the bone (see Figure 2.2). Mild thinning is called osteopenia, and severe thinning is called osteoporosis. Osteopenia occurs first and, if untreated, can progress to osteoporosis.

In the United States, 27.3 million women and 16.1 million men have osteopenia, and 8.2 million women and 2.0 million men have osteoporosis. In their lifetime, 1 in 3 women and 1 in 5 men will have an osteoporosis-related broken bone (fracture).

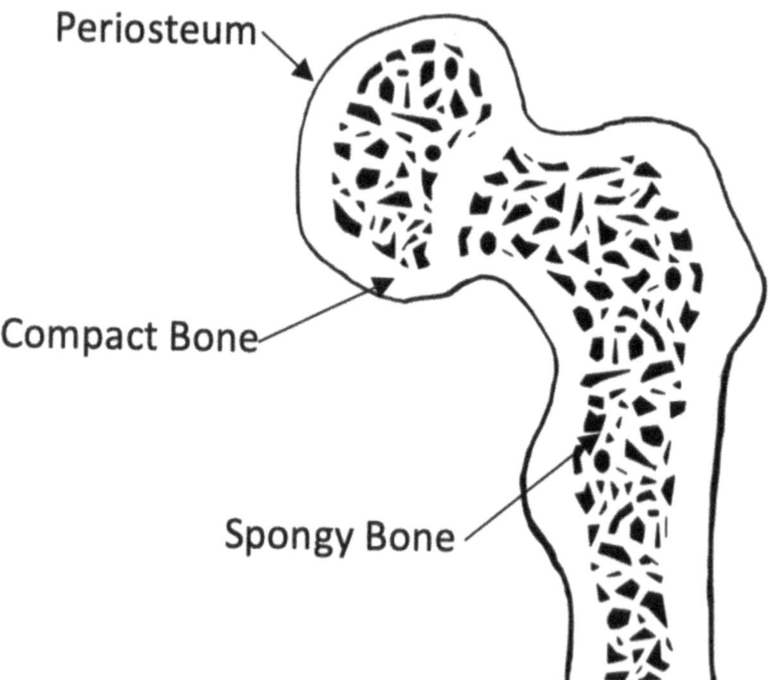

Figure 2.1. Anatomy of a bone.

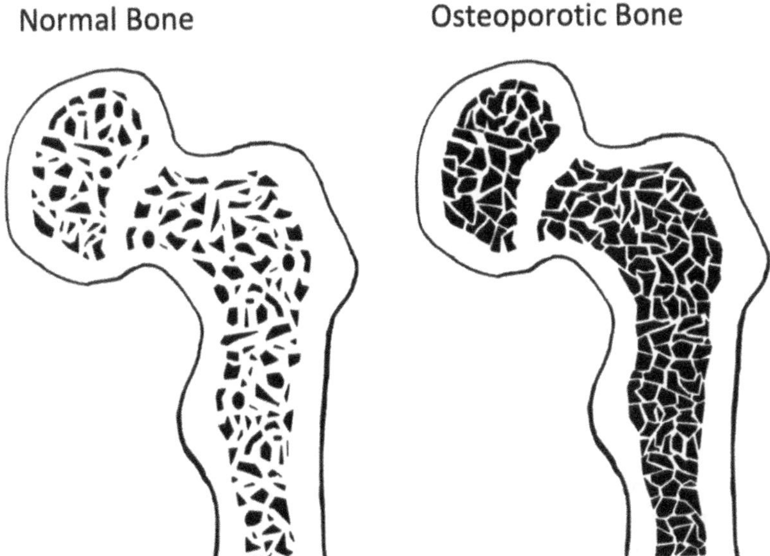

Figure 2.2. A comparison of normal bone and a bone with osteoporosis. The black areas represent open space.

Why Are Women Affected More Than Men?

Starting at around age thirty, men lose 1 percent of their bone mass per year for the rest of their lives. Women also start losing bone mass at 1 percent per year at age thirty, but during the ten years of perimenopause, women lose bone mass at a rate of 7 percent per year. After menopause, women go back to losing bone mass at 1 percent per year. It is this ten years of additional bone loss that make women so much more susceptible to osteoporosis and fractures. For some readers, it will be easier to make sense of these numbers if they see a graph of bone loss (see Figure 2.3). The graph shows the bone loss of men and women starting at the age of thirty through the age of ninety-five. At age thirty, men and women have 100 percent of their bone mass, and it declines from there. These numbers are for demonstration purposes. Individual variations such as genetics, body size, exercise, and diet can affect a person's bone density.

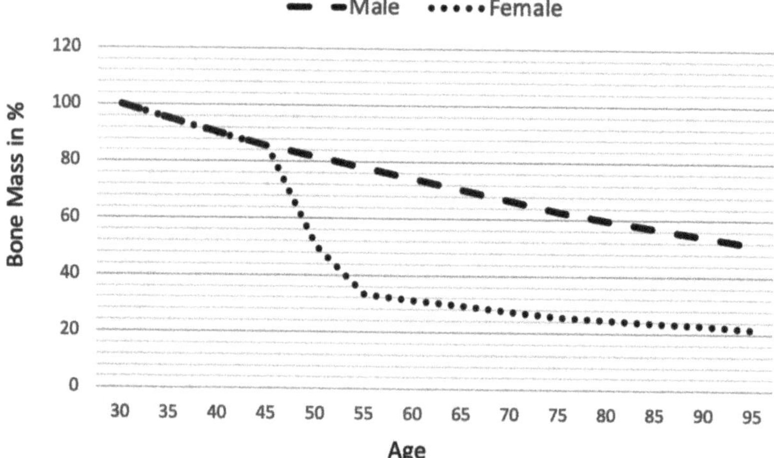

Figure 2.3. This graph is a representative example to compare the lifetime bone loss between males and females starting at age 30. Males are represented by the dashed line and females by the dotted line.

Diagnosis and Monitoring of Osteoporosis

A DEXA scan, also called a bone density scan, can be used to accurately measure an individual's bone density to see if their bones are stronger or weaker than average for their age. DEXA stands for dual-energy X-ray absorptiometry, and it uses two low-energy X-ray beams directed toward any bone to determine the bone mineral density. It does this by determining the amount of each beam that is absorbed by the bone. Typically, the DEXA scan measures the bones of your spine, hip, and long bone of the thigh (femur) and sometimes the forearm bone of the arm that you don't use to write with (nondominant radius).

As of 2020, the United States Preventative Services Task Force (USPSTF) recommends that all women get a bone density scan at age sixty-five because treatment of osteoporosis can moderately prevent fractures. The USPSTF also recommends that postmenopausal women at risk for osteoporosis be tested prior to age sixty-five. The task force did not find evidence of benefit or harm in treating men, so most physicians do not routinely check men for osteoporosis unless an individual has one or more risk factors.

The DEXA scan provides two scores for each bone tested: a Z score that compares your bone density to the average person your age, and a T score that compares your bone density to an average twenty-year-old. The Z score is interesting but not used for treatment or diagnostic purposes. The T score is used medically to determine if you have osteoporosis or osteopenia. A T score of greater than –1.0 is considered normal. A T score of –1.0 to –2.5 meets the criteria for osteopenia. A T score of less than –2.5 or an osteoporotic fracture meets the criteria for osteoporosis. An osteoporosis fracture includes femoral neck fractures (top of the thigh bone) and lumbar and thoracic vertebral fractures that occur when someone falls from a standing height.

Beatrice slipped in the bathroom, and she fell and broke her hip, specifically the femoral neck of the femur. Lynn coughed, heard something pop in her back, and then felt severe pain. Beatrice and Lynn both endured osteoporotic fractures and should be diagnosed with osteoporosis. Tom fell off his bike and broke his lumbar vertebrae. Bob was in a car accident and sustained a femoral neck fracture. Tom's and Bob's fractures are considered traumatic fractures due to accidents, not osteoporosis.

Everybody with osteoporosis should be treated with lifestyle modifications (exercise and vitamins) and medication. Currently, for people with osteopenia, a calculation is done to decide if you need to be treated with lifestyle modifications alone or with medication as well. If you have osteopenia, your doctor will calculate a FRAX score. The FRAX score calculation incorporates information about your age, sex, weight, height, prior fractures, family history of hip fractures, and bone density score of your femur as well as whether you smoke, are on steroid medications, have rheumatoid arthritis, and/or use alcohol daily. If the FRAX score predicts a 3 percent risk of hip fracture in the next ten years or a 10 percent risk of any fracture in the next ten years, then you should be treated with both lifestyle modifications and medication.

Some doctors also check C-telopeptide (CTX) levels to determine the rate of bone breakdown and propeptide type I collagen (P1NP) to assess new bone formation to determine whether treatment is indicated if you are young or male. Why? Young people with poor bone density may still be at low risk of fracture if they have good bone quality. Bone quality, however, cannot be routinely measured . . . yet! The CTX and P1NP values can also be followed to see if the medications that you are taking are working as expected.

All of the tips that follow you can do for yourself, and they also prevent osteopenia and help slow osteopenia from progressing to osteoporosis!

What You Can Do for Yourself

- Limit alcohol to less than seven drinks per week for women and less than ten drinks per week for men with a drink being 1.5 oz. of spirits at 40 percent alcohol by volume (abv), 12 oz. of beer at 5 percent abv, or 5 oz. wine at 12 percent abv.
- Avoid tobacco and vaping products. Both of these first two recommendations are easier said than done for some people, and if you are having trouble cutting down on your alcohol intake or stopping smoking, then talk with your doctor.
- Many people have heard that they should do weight-bearing exercises to help prevent or slow down the progression of bone loss but don't know what those include. The following are weight-bearing exercises that you would want to do for thirty minutes for four to five days of the week:
    - Brisk walking
    - Climbing stairs
    - Dancing
    - Hiking
    - Jogging
    - Jumping rope
    - Step aerobics
    - Tennis or other racquet sports
    - Yard work, like pushing a lawnmower or heavy gardening

    Then two to three days out of the week, the above weight-bearing exercises can be alternated with these weight-bearing exercises:
    - Elastic bands
    - Free weights
    - Weight machines
    - Push-ups
    - Squats
- By including simple exercises to improve balance, like standing on one foot, you can help prevent falls. Balance exercises work

by improving your reflexes and the more subtle awareness of your footing (proprioception), which can help you catch yourself if you start to fall.

- Take measures to limit falls, such as ensuring good lighting when moving around your home and unfamiliar areas (also see Chapter 25, "Home Safety").
- Ask your doctor how much vitamin D you should take. Most of my patients, who have a normal vitamin D level, are able to maintain a vitamin D level in the recommended range by taking 2,000 IU of Vitamin D3 per day. For patients that are deficient, higher doses are needed to get them caught up before they can be maintained on a lower dose.
  - Don't be surprised if you are vitamin D deficient. Most people need additional vitamin D, as we spend so much time indoors, and when we are outdoors in the sun, which is where we get most of our vitamin D, we are wearing sunscreen to prevent skin cancer. Sunscreen also blocks vitamin D absorption.
- Vitamin D works best to prevent fractures if it is taken with calcium (at least in women, as we know less about osteoporosis in men). This is likely because most people do not get enough calcium in their diets. The dietary recommendation is 1,200 to 1,500 mg/day.
  - There are some tips for taking supplemental calcium. If you take medication for heartburn, then you should take calcium citrate; otherwise, calcium carbonate is appropriate. Take your calcium with food to prevent constipation and bloating and 500 mg at a time to maximize absorption. If you need to take 1,000 mg, then split it into two doses that you can take throughout the day.
  - Calcium can also affect the absorption of iron, zinc, and magnesium as well as medications, including the following classes of medications: fluoroquinolone and tetracycline antibiotics, bisphosphonates, beta-blockers, and calcium channel blocker blood pressure medicines and anti-seizure medicines.

  - o The best way to avoid interactions is to take calcium two hours apart from your other medications. If that is too inconvenient, talk to your pharmacist to inquire about potential interactions of calcium with your medications.
- Some nutritionists are recommending adding K2 to vitamin D3 supplements. There are a few small studies that suggest K2 may help increase bone density when added to vitamin D3. It also impacts how your body clots blood, so before you start K2, be sure to talk with your doctor.

What Your Doctor Can Do

- Vitamin D can be found in many forms in the body, but your physician will specifically measure the 25-hydroxy type of vitamin D in your blood to assess your vitamin D level. Weighing the risks and benefits of various blood levels of vitamin D and the current literature, I recommend a goal blood level of vitamin D of 30 to 60 NG/ml.
- Advise you on how much vitamin D you should take. They can also discuss K2 with you.
- Review your daily intake of calcium and help you decide how much calcium you need to add to your diet.
- Order a bone density or DEXA scan.
- If you have osteopenia, your doctor can calculate a FRAX score to determine if you need medication.
- If you have osteoporosis or osteopenia with a FRAX score that recommends medication treatment, there are several options that your doctor can prescribe. Bisphosphonates, monoclonal antibodies, and parathyroid hormone analogs are described in detail below.

Details about Osteoporosis Medication

Bisphosphonates include medications such as alendronate (Fosamax®), ibandronate (Boniva®), risedronate (Actonel®), pamidronate (Aredia®), and zoledronic acid (Zometa®). They are used to prevent bone loss and are the most common medications used to treat osteoporosis. Evidence shows that bisphosphonates reduce the risk of fracture in postmenopausal women with osteoporosis. In healthy bone, bone is constantly breaking itself down with cells called osteoclasts and rebuilding healthy bone by cells called osteoblasts (see Figure 2.4). Bisphosphonates kill the osteoclasts, preventing bone loss. This group of medications is most commonly given in a pill form. The side effects include nausea, chest pain, hoarseness, and irritation of the esophagus. This can be avoided by sitting up (or standing) for thirty minutes after taking this medication.

Several of my patients have been afraid to take these medications because they heard about jawbone problems associated with the medication. This is a serious side effect called osteonecrosis. Osteonecrosis means the death of bone and usually occurs in the jaw. Fortunately, it is very rare and somewhat predictable. Ninety-five percent of the cases involved patients on chemotherapy or who were on steroids and had undergone a tooth extraction and/or had received intravenous bisphosphonates. This makes me feel confident prescribing oral medications for otherwise relatively healthy patients.

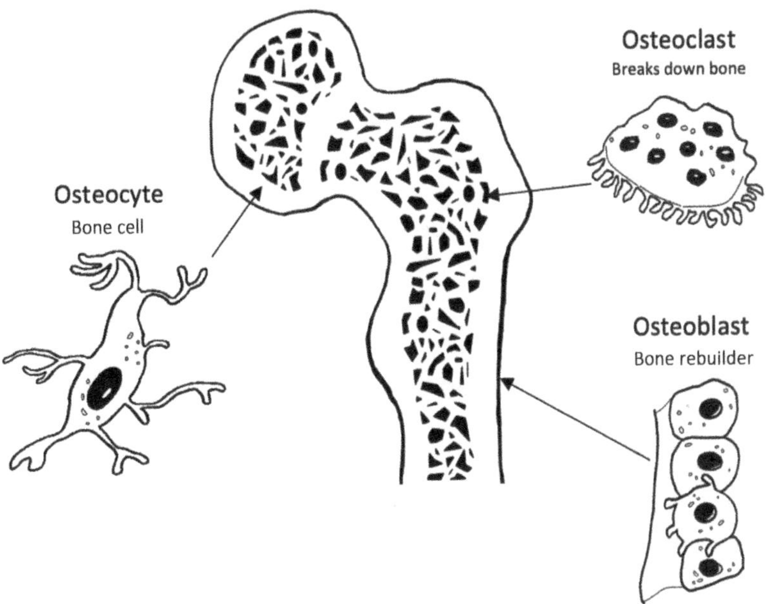

Figure 2.4. A bone showing different types of bone cells, where they live and how and they affect bone strength.

These medications should only be taken for five years. After five years, they increase the risk of a very unusual fracture called a chalk stick fracture of the femur or thigh bone. *Since many patients switch doctors, it is important for you to help your doctor keep track of how long you have been on one of these medications.*

There are two monoclonal antibody type medications used for osteoporosis called denosumab (Prolia®) and romosozumab (Evenity®). Denosumab also works to stop the osteoclasts, which are the cells that break down bone. It is more effective at increasing bone density than bisphosphonates in clinical trials. We don't yet know if that also means people who take these medications have fewer fractures than those on bisphosphonate. Serious side effects are similar to that of bisphosphonates. Romosozumab is very similar to denosumab and is recommended for patients with osteoporosis who have already had a fracture. It is dosed as a monthly shot.

The final category to be discussed is the parathyroid hormone analogs teriparatide (Forteo®) and abaloparatide (Tymlos®). These medications work by regulating calcium and phosphate metabolism in the bones and also in the kidneys. They increase bone mineral density by promoting new bone formation. Teriparatide is approved for both women and men! These medications are dosed through a daily injection. Side effects are usually mild, if any, and typically, patients are treated for two years, though they can safely be treated for longer. *Again, since many patients switch doctors, it is important for you to help your doctor keep track of how long you have been on one of these medications.*

Your doctor will help you decide which medication is best for you and what is the best sequence to take these medications since some of them have time limits.

Overcoming Osteoporosis

Let me tell you about George. While people with osteoporosis are usually women, George stands out in my mind because of his recent hip fracture. George is a spry ninety-year-old. Just one week prior to his hip fracture, he came into the office to see my partner for a routine visit. When he saw me in the hall, he announced: "Look what I can do!" Then, without holding on to the wall or counter, he did alternate leg lunges and then knelt down and stood back up without using his arms for support. I knew he was in good shape, but I was honestly impressed.

A week later, I heard that he had tripped over his cat and broke his hip. Knowing the poor statistical outcomes for the typical ninety-year-old after a hip fracture, I said to my partner, "I think he is going to do just fine!"

The next week, George came bounding into the office without needing a walker or a cane. He proudly showed off his surgical scar. Why was he not a statistic? He had been eating healthy, taking his vitamins, doing weight-bearing exercises, and his body was strong before the fracture. He healed quickly, did his physical therapy, and got back to life. This fracture led to a new diagnosis of osteoporosis. He is now on medication to prevent future fractures.

And then there was Josephine. I met Josephine for the first time on a gurney in the emergency department. She reported that she was in "good health," with no medical problems and on no medications. Her only problem was a fall and new hip pain. The high blood pressure flashing on the monitor behind her short, stout frame with a jolly belly and her right leg rotated outward told a different story. She had "avoided" health problems, only by avoiding all doctors for the past fifteen years. Now, at seventy, she was confronted with the reality of a hip fracture and at least a few other new diagnoses: osteoporosis, high blood pressure (hypertension), and obesity. I took care of her in the hospital, and her fracture got repaired. When it was time for her to leave the hospital, she still couldn't make it from the chair to the commode by herself, so she was discharged from the hospital to a rehabilitation facility to work on strength and independence. She desperately would have preferred to go home.

A year later, I saw Josephine volunteering in the hospital. She had lost forty pounds and wanted me to know that she was seeing a primary care doctor regularly, eating healthier, and exercising regularly. She also told me that her recovery was long, and it gave her time to think about how she wanted to spend her retirement. To cheer herself up during the long days in rehabilitation, she covered her walker in bright stickers, set health goals, and made a plan to return to the hospital as a volunteer.

She made it back home and is walking the hospital halls as a volunteer without a walker or cane. She even donated her walker back to the hospital, hoping to never use one again. Now every time she sees someone doing physical therapy in the hospital with her stickered walker, she yells, "Look, that one was mine!"

George and Josephine fell and broke their hips, but falls are not a sign of aging. Think about yourself as a youngster, as young as you can remember. Did you fall learning to walk? How many times did you fall off of your bike? Did you fall learning how to steal home plate or wrestling with your siblings? As a young adult, did you fall learning to ski or doing a karate kick? Did you trip running to greet a friend you hadn't seen in years? Were you walking your dog when it took off after a squirrel, only to leave you floating behind like a kite in the wind? Falling is not a sign of aging, but instead, it is a natural part of living. We fall at all stages of our lives because we are out there living them! Sometimes, gravity just gets the best of us.

Yes, bones get thinner with age, and you will fall as you are living your life, but they don't have to break, and broken bones don't have to negatively impact your quality of life. With the proper diet, adequate vitamins, and exercise to support bones and prevent dangerous falls, you can avoid osteoporosis. If you do sustain a fracture and you are taking care of your body, you will heal faster and resume your activities quicker than expected.

CHAPTER THREE
FALLS: I'M JUST RESTING . . . ON THE FLOOR

Age and Injury

Perhaps you remember a commercial that was aired every thirty minutes in the late 1980s/early 1990s. An older woman falls, and she lands on the floor in her bathroom beside her bathtub. She's wearing a blue-and-brown-striped dress and has one leg caught underneath her. A walker is tipped over next to her on the floor. She yells out, "I've fallen, and I can't get up." It was a catchphrase on a television commercial for Life Alert pendants. She presses the button, and a dispatcher responds, "We are sending help immediately, Mrs. Fletcher."

Actress Edith Fore became famous for playing Mrs. Fletcher, though the fall was actually performed by a stunt double. Maybe you remember that line, "I've fallen, and I can't get up," and repeated it jokingly or even chuckled at it when you were thirty years younger. Now, it may not seem quite as funny. Admit that you are a bit jealous of Mrs. Fletcher. Wouldn't it be nice to have a stunt double in real life for when you fall, just like she did?

When I moved from New York to Colorado, I was shocked at how fit everyone around me was (and is). I used to joke with my mother, "Ma, in New York, my friends would invite me for dinner. In Colorado, my friends ask if I want to run a marathon and then get some breakfast or hike a 14,000-foot mountain and grab lunch." I marveled at the athleticism all around me. Then, all of a sudden, my marathon-running, ultra-mountain-climbing, mountain peak-to-mountain peak hundred-mile bicycling friends hit their late fifties and sixties and started falling. They fell while they were just walking. Sometimes, they fell on ice, other times, they fell on loose rocks and gravel, and sometimes on uneven pavements. And they didn't just fall, they hurt themselves—broken bones, torn rotator cuffs, strained muscles, and injured backs. What about age makes people more likely to fall? What about age makes people more likely to get injured? How can it be prevented?

There are three main categories of elements that cause aging people to get injured when they fall, and they overlap like this Venn diagram (see Figure 3.1). Let's explore each of them separately.

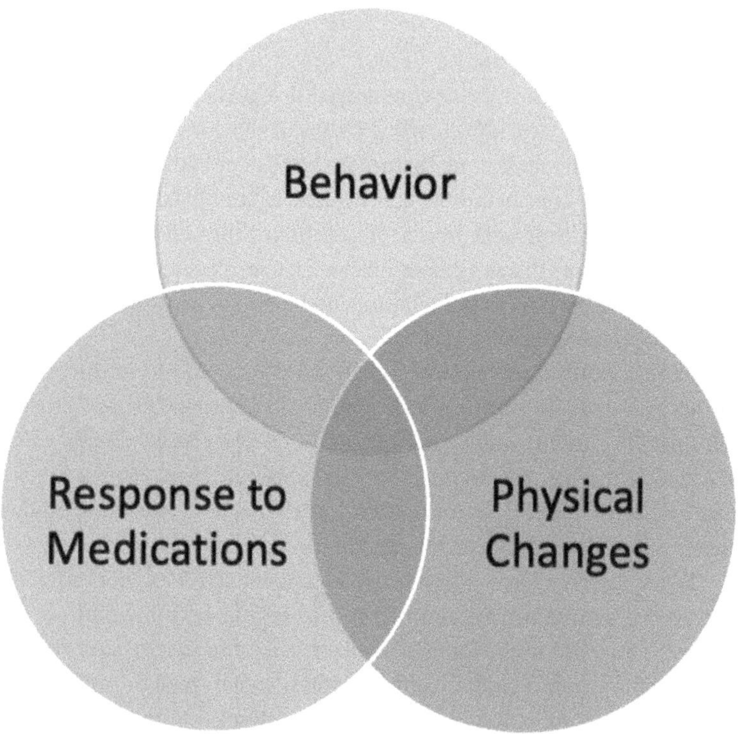

Figure 3.1. A Venn diagram demonstrating the causes of falls and how they overlap increasing fall risk.

Behavioral Causes

As people age, there are two potential behavioral changes that can occur. Patients who have fallen before or who are afraid of falling tend to lean forward and lower their bodies closer to the ground. They stand as if carrying themselves closer to the ground will reduce injury. In fact, this posture causes one's center of gravity to hover ahead of their body rather than over their feet, making them more likely to fall. Secondly, some patients, especially those with dementia and even mild cognitive impairment, become more impulsive (see Chapter 19). They jump up and move faster, not allowing time for their bodies to find their balance. They forget to lift their feet high enough, forget canes and walkers, and don't allow time for their blood pressure to equilibrate causing dizziness (see Chapter 14). My twenty-year-old niece is a top-trained chef and is on her feet all day. The muscles in her young, healthy legs and blood vessels pump the blood up from her legs to exactly where it needs to be in her body at all times as she moves around the kitchen at lightning speed. As people age, the walls of their blood vessels get filled with calcium and become stiff, so that when older people stand up, they are not able to squeeze the blood from the legs up to the brain, resulting in dizziness. Any quick movement doesn't give time for the body to compensate, and they fall.

Physical Changes

Arthritis causes stiffness and limits movement of the joints. Muscle loss (sarcopenia) reduces strength, making it harder to catch oneself if they become off-balance. Also, as people age, their reflexes greatly diminish. If I attempt to push my eighteen-year-old nephew over from behind, hard enough to knock him over, he will reach out his arms to catch himself and land with his hands close together near his face with his palms down. Eighty-year-olds fall more like an unconscious boxer or a felled tree. If I attempt to push my eighty-year-old neighbor from any direction (I never would), he will invariably hit his face first. His reflexes will not be fast enough to even attempt to lift his arms, and he will be left with a severely bruised face. One that I have sadly seen innumerable times in my career.

Let's go back to my nephew, who at eighteen also makes his aunt proud as I get to watch him on stage as he pursues his dreams in musical theatre. As an actor, singer, and dancer, he lifts women high into the air on a regular basis. If given the choice, would you trust an eighteen-year-old to lift you off the ground over a seventy-five-year-old? What if I told you that the seventy-five-year-old was also an actor, singer, and dancer? First, we must confront our biases about age. If the seventy-five-year-old has assessed, addressed, and compensated for changes to his body over the years, he is likely just as reliable as the eighteen-year-old in his lifts!

Diminished vision is another physical change that can result in falls if not addressed. As we age, some experience impaired visual acuity, depth perception, and ability to detect contrast between objects and/or limited vision in the dark. Hearing and other inner ear (vestibular) impairments affect balance by altering perception of one's location relative to their environment. It becomes harder to tell, for example, if you are leaning too far backward or too far forward. Feet are also less sensitive, so it can be more difficult to feel slopes and bumps in the terrain that your balance and reflexes need to accommodate to avoid falls. There is also some evidence to suggest that poor nutrition, which is more prevalent in the elderly, increases one's risk for falls. All of these physical changes are just a natural part of the aging process. Any additional illness would only make the risks of falling higher.

Response to Medications

Lastly, older people tend to be on more medications to manage a growing list of medical ailments that they have accumulated throughout their long lives. Any medication that can make the brain a bit foggy can contribute to falls. Even medication as simple as diphenhydramine (Benadryl®) for allergies, sedatives for insomnia, opioids for pain, benzodiazepines for anxiety, muscle relaxants, and alcohol can greatly increase the risk of falls. While you may have taken these medications your entire life, as you age, the side effects become greater. Also, any medication or medical condition like benign prostate hyperplasia (BPH) that causes you to urinate at night or that lowers your blood pressure increases your risk of falls. (See more on medications in Chapter 17.)

Go to Your Doctor

If you have fallen, your doctor will inquire about injuries and whether or not you have hit your head. He or she will take your vital signs. Then the physical exam will be very much tailored to you as an individual. Your doctor may repeat your blood pressure and pulse in various positions, including lying down and sitting and standing up. Your physical exam might include testing of your vision and hearing. The exam may test your gait, your balance, your strength, and your nerves. You might not even notice the doctor do this part of the exam, as we are very subtle about watching you enter the exam room and move from the chair to the exam table. The exam may include a closer look at certain joints, the bottoms of your feet, and your skin for injury. Sometimes, bloodwork is indicated. Sometimes, patients need additional cardiac testing to look for abnormal heart rhythms, X-rays for arthritis or broken bones, or EEGs to look for seizure activity. The diagnostic workup is really based on the judgment of your doctor, and all of these tests are by no means required, nor are they helpful for many patients. I just want to give you an idea as to what you might encounter.

Risks of Falls

With falls come some dreaded risks. Most patients fear hip fractures for themselves or their older relatives and friends. The one-year mortality rate of hip fracture is fairly high. Though you can die from a hip fracture itself, that is rare. Most people end up dying from the consequence of decreased mobility in the months following the injury. After hip fractures, patients tend to move less and lie in bed more. They develop pressure ulcers or bedsores (decubitus ulcers) on their buttocks that become infected. If you stay in a bed for long periods of time, the bottoms of your lungs begin to collapse (atelectasis). The collapsed lung tissue becomes a warm, moist place for bacteria to grow, and patients develop pneumonia. It's these infections that often lead to death.

Sometimes when patients fall, they land on furniture, breaking ribs. Broken ribs are also very dangerous because the pain causes splinting, and patients don't want to take deep breaths. Shallow breaths lead to collapsed lungs and, just like we discussed, pneumonia follows.

What if a patient falls and lies on the floor for six or eight hours before someone finds them? Then, in addition to the cuts and bruises, patients can develop bedsores, muscle breakdown, and kidney failure. While lying on the ground, bedsores form on all of the bony parts of the body that are in contact with the floor. It is not uncommon to see bedsores develop on a person's forehead, shoulder, elbow, knee, and ankle. Muscles then break down while lying on the ground, causing extra protein to float around in the blood. This is called rhabdomyolysis. These proteins can then clog the kidneys and cause kidney failure. All of these conditions worsen the longer a person is on the ground without water, getting dehydrated. This didn't happen to Mrs. Fletcher, who we learned about at the beginning of the chapter, because she was able to call for help right away with her Life Alert pendant.

The other thing that doctors worry about when a patient falls is bleeding in the brain. It is natural for our brains to shrink with age. This allows the brain more room to rattle within the skull when someone falls. Blood vessels that bridge between the brain and the skulls get pulled and stretched when the brain shakes during a fall. This increases the risk of a torn blood vessel and bleeding around the brain called a subdural hematoma (see Figure 3.2). When torn, these can be minor, causing no symptoms, or more severe, causing stroke-like symptoms or lead to someone's death.

While this may sound like a terribly sad list of consequences from falls, there is also hope in that there are many, many things that you can do to avoid falls and injury.

What You Can Do for Yourself

- Footwear—Thin, hard-sole shoes are the best for improving balance and reducing falls, though perceived as less comfortable than thick, soft shoes. Athletic shoes or sneakers are also a great choice and much better than barefoot, high heels, stockings, or slippers.
- Turn on the lights—Give yourself the best chance of seeing things that you might trip on . . . like the ever-so-quiet sneaky cat. Does the bathroom have a night light? Why not put them throughout your home? Ours have movement detectors built in so that they only come on when needed.

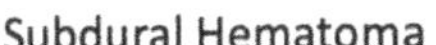

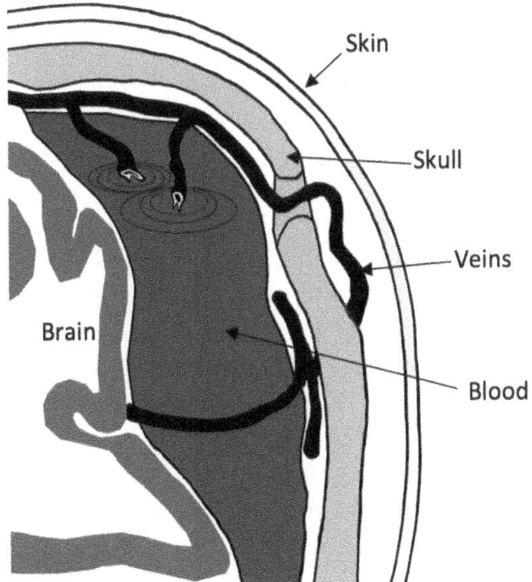

Figure 3.2. A subdural hematoma. A smaller aged brain moves in the skull, tearing veins that span the distance from the brain to the skull. The bleeding then gets trapped between the brain and the skull resulting in a subdural hematoma.

- Wear sensory aids—Make sure your glasses are the right prescription and that your hearing aids have batteries, and you wear them.
- Clear your paths—Identify direct paths from the bed to the bathroom, your favorite chair to the bathroom, the kitchen to the living room, and then widen and unclutter the paths. This may require removing furniture and tying up or tucking extension cords behind furniture.
- Safety devices—Consider handrails going up all stairs inside and outside your home, in the shower and bathtub, next to the bed, and around the toilet. Consider a shower chair. Raise the toilet seat. If you need a cane or walker, use one. Many Coloradoans use a hiking pole instead of a cane to maintain their youthful appearance since everyone uses them to descend steep mountain trails.

- Remove hazards—Eliminate throw rugs and mats that can easily be tripped on. Go with wall-to-wall carpeting or just plain flooring. Empty high cabinets in the kitchen to avoid reaching and climbing.
- Exercise—You want to focus on balance, posture, and thigh strength starting in your fifties. Some people benefit from working with a trainer or physical therapist. Some people prefer to join a yoga or other balance fitness class. Others practice standing on one foot while brushing their teeth, heel lifts where you stand on the ball of your feet, tandem walking (heel to toe in a straight line), and standing from a deep-seated position. To do this, sit on the bottom step of a set of stairs or curb and simply stand up . . . as many times as you can. Don't forget to make sure that you use good form—don't let your knees pass your toes, stand straight up aiming your head at the ceiling the entire time, and, ideally, don't use your hands to help.
- Stay hydrated—Water is your friend. Caffeine and alcohol are very dehydrating.
- Review your medication list with your physician at your physical—If certain pills, like diuretics or water pills, make you get up at night to urinate, ask your doctor if you can take them earlier in the day.

If you have fallen, there are things you can do to help yourself.

- If your risk of falling is high, have an alert button accessible or a phone in your pocket so that if you do fall again, you can call for help and don't have to lie on the floor for an extended period of time.
- After an injury, while you are less mobile, use an incentive spirometer inhalation device or just take a deep breath and hold for three seconds. Do this ten to twelve times an hour while you are awake.
- If you are on the floor or in bed recovering, rotate your body position every two hours to avoid bedsores.

- Even if you didn't injure yourself, request physical therapy to help with strength and balance to prevent future falls. If you did injure yourself, the exercises would help restore you to your best level of functioning much more quickly than if you try to do it on your own.
- See your doctor. Your injuries may be more severe than you thought.

What Your Doctor Can Do

- Assess you for injury.
- Order X-rays and CT scans to look for broken bones and bleeding.
- Check bloodwork to rule out rhabdomyolysis and kidney failure.
- Order physical therapy to help prevent future falls.
- Treat any skin wounds.
- Review your medications with you, including over-the-counter medications and supplements to prevent future falls.

Prevention

Our practice is across from a small city park. A few times a year, we hire a physical therapist named Shae to teach classes on balance training at the park. She is very talented, and the patients love her. I love that patients are learning the skills that they need to prevent falls while building a small community. There are too many lonely seniors in the world. Each event we host is like a small reunion where people gather who recognize each other from their earlier lives, their place of worship, community groups, the waiting room, or other events we have hosted.

One of our patients, Barbara, wanted me to know that she had fallen. She was standing on carpet and, with one foot, stepped out onto a hardwood floor. The floor was much more slippery than she had expected, and she fell. She was so elated to report, "Dr. Guerrasio, I fell, and I didn't get hurt! I know it was because of that balance class that I didn't get hurt. As I was going down, I landed differently because of everything I had been taught, and I didn't get hurt!" I'm sure there have been fewer falls because of her classes, but I never hear about those!

There are so many ways to prevent falls and injuries. I am often disheartened to see patients take the shortcuts and skip these recommendations. I hate seeing people suffer. If you have had an embolic stroke (clotting stroke rather than a bleeding stroke), your doctor likely prescribed you an aspirin a day. Out of fear of another stroke, you faithfully take that aspirin every day. The nine suggestions listed under the section "What You Can Do" are as effective at reducing falls as an aspirin a day is at reducing subsequent strokes. You have just as much control over whether you have a fall as people who have had a stroke have over having a second stroke! You likely wouldn't give a daily aspirin a second thought; don't give these tips a second thought either. You are in the driver's seat with this one.

CHAPTER FOUR
SKIN CARE: SMILE THROUGH THE WRINKLES

Mirror Tricks

As you might imagine, I get my lighthearted nature and sense of humor from my parents, and they are quite a pair. My mother has her memorable moments, like the time she looked in the mirror and asked me, "Who is that old lady staring back at me?" Even in her seventies, she still feels very much like her young teenage self. She often says she feels the same as when she first met my father at age sixteen.

One of the first visible signs of aging is our skin. How well are you taking care of your skin to reduce wrinkles, age spots, loose skin, and skin cancers? Remember, no matter how old you are when you get your hands on this book, it is never too late to adjust the trajectory of your aging process. You get to pick and choose your priorities and decide what is important to you and where you want to invest your time, money, and energy. Fortunately, taking care of your skin is one of the simplest things to do.

What You Can Do for Yourself

- Protect your skin from the sun every day. Whether spending a day at the beach or running errands, sun protection is essential. You can protect your skin by seeking shade, covering up with clothing, and/or using sunscreen that is broad-spectrum,

SPF 30 (or higher), and water-resistant. You should apply sunscreen every day to all skin that is not covered by clothing.

- Apply self-tanner rather than get a tan. Every time you get a tan, you prematurely age your skin. This holds true if you get a tan from the sun, a tanning bed, or other indoor tanning equipment. All emit harmful ultraviolet (UV) rays that accelerate how quickly your skin ages and are not protective. Self-tanner does not do the same damage.
- If you smoke, ask for help to quit. Smoking greatly speeds up how quickly skin ages. It causes wrinkles and a dull, sallow complexion. Wrinkles concentrate around the mouth from drawing on the cigarette, cigar, pipe, or joint and around the eyes from squinting due to the smoke.
- Avoid repetitive facial expressions. Remember when you frowned as a child or stuck your tongue out at your siblings and your mom said, "Keep making that face and it will freeze that way!" Once again . . . mom was right. When you make a facial expression, you contract the underlying muscles. If you repeatedly contract the same muscles for many years, the overlying skin lines become permanent. That is why sunglasses are recommended. Wearing sunglasses can help reduce wrinkle lines caused by squinting. However, I personally make an exception when it comes to smiling. Smiling to me is worth every wrinkle!
- Eat a healthy, well-balanced diet. Findings from a few studies suggest that eating plenty of fresh fruits and vegetables may help prevent damage that leads to premature skin aging. Findings from research studies also suggest that a diet containing lots of sugar or other refined carbohydrates can accelerate aging.
- Stay well hydrated. Dehydration, especially from alcohol, deepens wrinkles and makes skin look withered. Hydration keeps your skin looking bright and vital by maintaining the skin's elasticity. Alcohol also depletes the body of vitamin A, which plays an important role in skin firmness.
- Schedule an annual skin check. Last but not least, annual skin checks with a dermatologist preferably or at least a primary

care physician are essential. Skin cancers are common and easily removed if caught early. If ignored, they can be very destructive, cosmetically and functionally, depending on where they are located. Go to a professional with experience, if possible, as skin cancers look very different on each individual depending on the location on the body, their skin tone, skin color, age, and so on. If the doctor does not look at every inch of your skin, pick another doctor.

What Your Doctor Can Do

- Differentiate dangerous skin lesions from those that are not dangerous.
- Biopsy and remove concerning skin lesions.
- Recommend which products are best for your skin type, if your skin needs more than what I have recommended, or provide prescription-strength creams and lotions.
- Provide Botox® injections (see below for more).

A Sample Skin Routine

Some people ask me to recommend a skin-care routine, so I would like to offer one. In the morning, wash your face daily with a gentle face wash such as Dove®, Cetaphil®, or CeraVe®. Then, regardless of the season, apply a moisturizer with sunscreen every morning to your face, neck, chest, and the tops of your hands. The sunscreen should contain at least SPF 30+ with zinc and/or titanium. Zinc and titanium serve as a physical sunscreen that physically blocks against UV light, allowing it to bounce off. Chemical sunscreens turn UV light into heat. A combination of a chemical and physical sunscreen is best. Since I am often asked, I personally use ELTA MD® tinted sunscreen on my face and the tops of my hands every day.

For the most ambitious skin-care takers, you can also apply a daily antioxidant serum containing vitamins C and E to bare skin after washing and before applying sunscreen (e.g., Skinceuticals®, Ferulic CE®, etc.) and take a daily oral antioxidant containing niacinamide (e.g., Heliocare®).

In the evening, wash your face daily with a gentle face wash such as Dove®, Cetaphil®, or CeraVe®. Apply an over-the-counter moisturizer containing retinol or a prescription-strength retinoid followed by a gentle moisturizing lotion with ceramides and hyaluronic acid (e.g., CeraVe PM®) several nights per week. Don't tell anyone, but I put a touch of retinol on top of my hands every night too to prevent old-age spots after putting some on my face, followed by a thin coat of CeraVe PM®. No spots yet!

Retinoids are derived from vitamin A, disperse pigment helping to prevent brown spots, normalize keratinocyte turnover unclogging pores, prevent acne, shrink pores, and treat precancerous skin changes. Retinoids also build collagen to prevent fine wrinkles. Retinoids, however, can be very drying and make the skin more sensitive to the sun, so if you choose to use a retinoid, you must be equally committed to sunscreen and moisturizing. Retinoids work best if used daily.

Spend Wisely on Skin Products

May I impart a few words to the wise? Aside from the treatments discussed, paying extra for exotic vitamins in skin creams that promise to erase fine lines and prevent wrinkles will get you little more than an empty wallet. Very, very few are actually effective in preventing or reversing skin damage. This is because the molecules in the creams are either too large to be absorbed by the skin or the creams contain antioxidants at concentrations that are too low to be effective. For example, collagen is a huge molecule that is not absorbed into the skin. So, it comes as no surprise that there is no strong evidence for the clinical efficacy of either oral or topical collagen. Only selenium, vitamin E, and vitamin C have been proven to decrease the effects of sun on the skin and actually prevent further damage.

Botox® and fillers are also used cosmetically. Studies have shown that they make you look younger, not just because it makes wrinkle lines less deep, but because they increase confidence, and you present a happier face. Another option might just be to smile more. Smiling alone makes people look more attractive and younger while at the same time relieving stress and elevating our moods. Did you know that smiling also lowers your blood pressure, controls your heart rate, and boosts your immune system? Next time you are with others, smile and see how many other people smile too! Smiling releases "feel good" hormones, such as endorphins and serotonin, into our bloodstreams. Share that good feeling and your beauty by smiling more. (More on these hormones in Chapter 22.)

Unwanted Hair Removal

Have you ever thought, "Why is hair growing where I *don't* want it and not where I *do* want it?" For those of us who are sprouting hairs in unexpected and unwanted places, may I suggest a good pair of tweezers or nose-hair/ear-hair trimmers? You will also need an honest friend with good vision to point out the ones you can't see. Other than that, the vast majority of skin care is within your control and takes but minutes a day.

CHAPTER FIVE
HAIR LOSS: YOUR FAVORITE HAIRS ARE VANISHING

When the Salons Closed

Apart from the Biblical story of Samson and Delilah, I truly didn't realize how important hair was until salons were closed during the COVID-19 pandemic. Yes, my patients wanted to go to see their friends and family. They wanted to go to the grocery store. They wanted to return to their places of worship. But the most common questions I got asked were, "When can I get my hair done?" and "Is it safe to return to the salon?"

After hearing those questions over and over, it reinforced that hair is very important to people. I have yet to meet a person that isn't bothered, even a little, when they notice the first signs of hair loss. What most people don't realize is that age-related baldness and thinning hair can affect men *and* women.

Men typically lose the hair at the crown, or very top, of the head first and then across the entire dome while at the same time experiencing a receding hairline as the hairs in the front run fleeting backward away from the forehead temples. Women tend to lose hair from the center part, and it spreads to the sides. Thinning at the temples can also occur (see Figure 5.1).

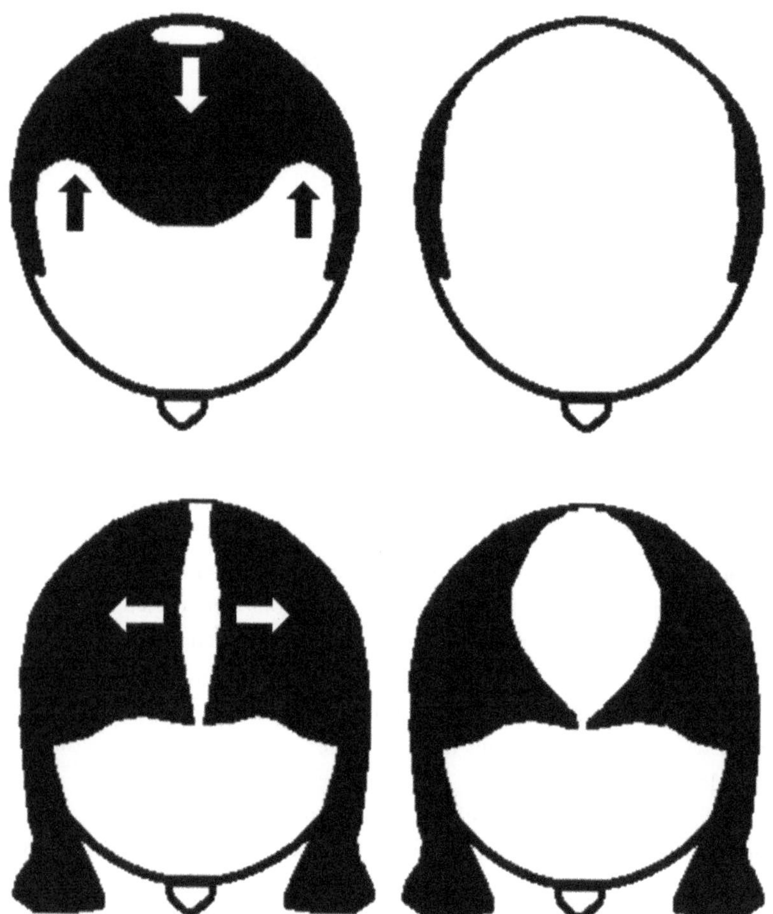

Figure 5.1. A comparison of male and female hair loss.

Male-Pattern Baldness

The medical name for age-related male-pattern baldness is male androgenetic alopecia, and it can start any time after puberty and progresses with age. It is hereditary and is related to the increase and fluctuations of the hormone dihydrotestosterone (DHT), a chemical that is formed when the body breaks down testosterone. If you look at all of your male friends or even brothers in the same family, you will notice that the severity of baldness is quite variable and that some men initially lose more hair in the front while others lose more on the top of their heads.

Multiple studies have shown a relationship between cardiovascular disease and hair loss. Patients with male-pattern baldness are also more likely to have high blood pressure (hypertension), be overweight, have high cholesterol (hyperlipidemia), and have diabetes mellitus. A correlation with prostate cancer has been investigated but has not been clearly established.

Female-Pattern Hair Loss

The medical name for age-related female-related baldness and thinning hair is female-pattern hair loss as some of the hair loss might be related to androgenetic (hormone-related) alopecia while others may not. Unfortunately, female-pattern hair loss is not as well understood as male-pattern baldness. It commonly occurs after menopause and progresses with age. Our understanding of how hormones and genetics affect female-pattern hair loss is incomplete.

Women with female-pattern hair loss are more likely than men to suffer from distress related to their hair loss, including negative body images, poor self-esteem, and less-satisfying quality of life. They are also more likely to be diagnosed with ovarian and adrenal tumors, adrenal gland enlargement (adrenal hyperplasia), high blood pressure (hypertension), diabetes, and cardiovascular disease.

What You Can Do for Yourself

- If you have female- or male-pattern baldness, let this serve as encouragement to meet with your doctor for your annual physical and regular check-ups and to manage any underlying chronic diseases. Hair loss may be an early sign of other diseases to come, and you want to avoid any unnecessary medical diseases or complications.
- Topical minoxidil is available over the counter in concentrations of 2 percent and 5 percent. I would recommend either the 5 percent solution or 5 percent foam. The foam is less likely to irritate the skin, but I consider both to be safe and well-tolerated by my patients.

- Medications for hair loss work best if used before the hair is gone, so start them as soon as you see thinning. Use them on the scalp, not the hair. There may be some initial hair loss during the first two months of use, before growth is established.
- Low-level laser light therapy (LLLT) can increase hair density, although the duration of effect is still being studied.
- Buy yourself fancy scarves, wigs, toupees, or just love your bald head!

What Your Doctor Can Do

- Confirm the diagnosis, as there are many other types of baldness.
- Review treatment options
  - Finasteride (Propecia) works by blocking the breakdown of testosterone to DHT by about 60 percent. When measured over a two-year period, approximately two-thirds of men have hair growth, and one-third stop losing hair but don't show any increase in scalp coverage. This treatment is less well studied in women.
  - For women, spironolactone can block male hormones and help stimulate hair regrowth.
  - Follicular unit transplantation and follicular unit extraction have come a long way over the past several decades, and I am amazed by the results! Hair is taken from non-balding areas of the head and moved to balding areas (and even to make beards!). The implanted hairs grow and turn gray, just like normal hair. Baldness, though, may continue to occur around the transplanted area, requiring recurrent surgeries to fill in the newly bare areas.
- Research is currently being done on prostaglandin topical medications, antifungal shampoos, and camouflaging agents such as sprays, lotions, and platelet-rich plasma. For women, mesotherapy, microneedling, topical estrogens, and supplements have yet to show any clear benefits, though supplements such as iron, biotin, ginseng, saw palmetto, green tea, and caffeine have been touted for hair regrowth or at least thickening

of the current hairs. Biotin does thicken hair. I have not seen improvements with the rest.

- Identify and help you manage any diseases associated with baldness.

Through the Eyes of Children

If only we can see baldness through the eyes of our children and grandchildren. If you are their parent or grandparent and you are bald or have thinning hair, it is just one feature of you, like your eye color or your height. They never stop to think, "Oh look, my dad is bald" or "Grandma's hair is thin." In their minds, they just feel lucky that you belong to them. But if you prefer to have a warmer head or skin without the risk of increased sun exposure and skin cancer, now you know what can be done. These are the tools that are currently available in the toolbox, with more on their way in the years to come.

CHAPTER SIX
ORAL HEALTH: OPEN WIDE!

Oral Hygiene

Some people are better rule followers than others. Some people are more organized. Some people invest more time in their health and wellness. These are likely the same folks that brush their teeth multiple times a day and floss daily rather than the day before their dentist appointment and after the occasional corn on the cob leaves some annoying kernel between their teeth. But good oral hygiene isn't just important because your dentist says you should do it.

Perhaps you remember Lucy's famous lines, "Ugh, I've been kissed by a dog! I have dog germs!" The dog Snoopy likely had dog breath and a mouth full of bacteria. What Lucy didn't realize when she requested a kiss from Schroeder without hesitation was that human mouths are also full of bacteria.

How Oral Health Affects Your Body

When people maintain good oral hygiene and are otherwise healthy, their body's immune system keeps their oral bacteria contained and prevents the bacteria from wreaking havoc on the rest of their bodies. It will likely come as no surprise that if you didn't brush your teeth you would end up with tooth decay, leading to cavities and gum diseases like gingivitis and periodontitis. But did you realize that poor oral health can lead to diseases in other parts of your body? And conversely, diseases in your body can lead to worsening oral health.

I had a patient come to my office complaining of severe fatigue. I asked him if he had any other symptoms, and he reported none. I then proceeded to ask him a series of questions from head to toe, just to make sure we weren't missing anything. "Do you have headaches? Sinus congestion? Problems with your ears?" His responses were all no until I got to his mouth. He denied problems chewing but did say that one of his teeth was bothering him a bit. After examining his mouth, I encouraged him to make an appointment with his dentist.

When he returned two weeks later for his physical, he announced that his fatigue was completely gone! The dentist had found an abscess under a cracked tooth. She drained the abscess, treated him with antibiotics, and took care of the tooth. And so went his total body fatigue.

I am so grateful for dentists who have skills and oral instruments that physicians do not. But I do regret that dentistry is treated separately from general medical care. Routine oral health care is no less important than routine health care that you get from your doctor. Everything that happens in the mouth affects your overall health. Here are just some of the most common risks of poor oral health.

If a patient has a lot of bacteria in their mouth and they develop an abscess or a cut in their mouth, the bacteria can enter into the bloodstream. This is called bacteremia. Patients with bacteremia have infection throughout their body because it is circulating in the blood to all of the organs and limbs. This can lead to a life-threatening condition called sepsis. Bacteremia can also be difficult to treat, requiring weeks of intravenous antibiotics and even surgery, if the bacteria attach themselves to the patient's heart valves (endocarditis) or artificial (prosthetic) joints.

While the connection between gum disease and cardiovascular disease is not entirely understood, patients with a lot of inflammation in their mouth are more likely to have heart attacks (myocardial infarctions), clogged arteries (atherosclerosis), and strokes (cerebral vascular accidents).

If your mouth is full of bacteria and fungi, it can be inhaled (aspirated) into the lungs. Aspiration can also occur when people swallow and saliva ends up in their lungs instead of in their esophagus and stomach. This can occur if throat muscles are weak or they swallow incorrectly. Once bacteria or fungi get into the lungs, they can cause a host of problems, including pneumonia, pneumonitis, or bronchiectasis. Pneumonia is a lung infection. Pneumonitis is thought as more of chemical irritation from saliva being so different than the moisture in the lungs. It then causes inflammation of the lungs that leads to scarring rather than outright infection. Bronchiectasis is a dilation of the airways in the lungs that increases the risk of infection, and these dilated airways fill with mucus.

Gum disease, like any infection, doesn't cause diabetes, but it definitely makes diabetes harder to treat. Gum disease raises blood sugar and makes blood sugars more difficult to regulate. Gum disease also can worsen the inflammation in a patient's lungs, worsening asthma and chronic obstructive pulmonary disease (COPD).

Medical Problems that Make Oral Health Worse

While we are on the topic of oral health, it is equally important to be aware of medical problems that can make oral health worse. High blood sugars feed bacteria, increasing the number of bacterial colonies in your mouth and throat. High blood sugars also increase your risk of other types of infections, including viral and fungal infections. With more bacteria, virus particles, and fungi in your mouth, you are more likely to inhale these invaders into your lungs. Diabetes also reduces the body's immune system, increasing the frequency and severity of gum disease.

Osteoporosis itself, separate from medication side effects, causes bone loss, and it is also linked with periodontal bone loss and tooth loss.

Cognitive decline makes it harder to maintain oral hygiene, and patients are more likely to develop oral diseases.

Cigarettes, e-cigarettes, cigars, pipes, marijuana, and alcohol all increase the risk of oral and throat cancers, some through toxins and others through the HPV virus.

HIV infection impairs the body's immune system, increasing the likelihood of infection throughout the body, including the mouth. People with HIV can develop viral ulcers, aphthous ulcers, fungal infections, more severe gum disease, and tooth decay.

Diseases that decrease saliva include an autoimmune disease called Sjögren's syndrome, rheumatoid arthritis, and certain cancers. Sjögren's syndrome causes dry eyes and mouth. Rheumatoid arthritis is better known for the hand arthritis that it causes, but it has many other symptoms, including dry mouth. Treatments, including radiation to the head and neck, decongestants, antihistamines, painkillers, and water pills (diuretics), all can cause dry mouth. Saliva is needed to neutralize the acid produced by bacteria, and without saliva to wash away bacteria and bits of food, oral diseases can worsen.

Some medications, like inhaled steroid medications, can lead to oral fungal infections. This is why you should rinse your mouth out with water after using inhaled steroids.

What You Can Do

- See your dentist and dental hygienist semi-annually for a cleaning.
- Take heed when the dentist gently reminds you to maintain oral hygiene. They will likely tell you to brush your teeth at least twice a day with a soft-bristled brush using fluoride toothpaste. Electric toothbrushes reduce plaque and gingivitis more than manual toothbrushes, with oscillating or rotating toothbrushes preferred over vibrating toothbrushes.
- Floss daily and rinse your mouth after. Water flosser devices are better than nothing, but good old-fashioned floss is better at removing bacteria from teeth and gums.
- Mouthwash is not a necessary part of oral health unless you are not otherwise able to clean your mouth well. It is not a substitute for brushing or flossing.
- Eat a healthy diet and limit food with added sugars.
- Avoid tobacco and marijuana, and limit alcohol.
- Replace your toothbrush when the bristles start to splay.
- Also, be sure your dentist has an updated medication list and knows your health history.
- Be sure to take care of any underlying chronic health conditions.
- If you have multiple medical problems to address, ask your doctor to help you prioritize how you approach your health. Don't leave your teeth for last . . . sometimes, they need to be fixed first!

What Your Dentist Will Do

- I have no idea. I'm not a dentist. But my dentist friends say they can do all of the following and more!
- Remove tooth decay, fill cavities, repair fractured teeth.
- Patch receding gums.
- Diagnose and treat gum, lip, and other oral diseases.
- Assess for oral cancers and biopsy abnormal lesions.
- Assess and treat problems with the jaw, including the main joints of the jaw that are just in front of the ears called the temporomandibular joints.
- Remove teeth.
- Fit partials, dentures, and implants.
- Repair facial cuts by stitching them up.

When to Call Your Dentist

Call your dentist if you notice:

- Gums that bleed during brushing and flossing
- Red, swollen, or tender gums
- Gums that have pulled away from your teeth
- Persistent bad breath
- Pus between your teeth and gums
- Loose or separating teeth
- A change in the way your teeth fit together when you bite
- A change in the fit of partial dentures or dentures

Looking Forward

I frequently see complications from delays in dental care. Hank had a cracked tooth that should have been a simple root canal, but he waited too long to see his dentist, and now he requires a full tooth extraction and implant instead.

Sue had some pain at the base of one of her molars. Less than excited about going to the dentist, she hoped it would just go away. Instead, she developed an oral abscess that spread to the blood (bacteremia) and then to her five-year-old artificial (prosthetic) right knee. The bacteria, as it always does, stuck hard and fast to the metal, and the only way to rid her body of the infection was to remove the prosthesis, surgically place an antibiotic-coated block (spacer), and give her six weeks of IV antibiotics. After the antibiotics were complete, a new artificial knee could be implanted.

Dwayne had a seemingly innocuous tooth broken at the gumline that led to bacteremia and a heart valve infection, open-heart surgery, and six months of cardiac rehabilitation before an eventual full recovery.

In most cases, I suspect delays in dental care are related to cost and poor insurance coverage, which may not be preventable. However, if at all possible, I promise, prevention will save you thousands of dollars and tons of heartache in the long run!

One last thought before we move on. Are you familiar with tooth fairy folklore? It is thought to have originated in Northern Europe around the year 1200 CE (AD), in which a fairy would come and pay a child for their first lost tooth. In the United States, it has expanded to include traditions of placing all lost teeth under one's pillow for a monetary gift from the tooth fairy. However, I remain deeply disappointed at the tooth fairy. Losing a tooth is more traumatic as an adult than as a child, and yet the tooth fairy abandons us beyond the age of eight.

Shall we start a new tradition right now? Every time you go to the dentist and lose even a part of a tooth from a cavity repair, root canal, or extraction, treat yourself to something small and special as if being visited by the tooth fairy. Don't ask your dentist for the remaining tooth to put under your pillow, just reward yourself for overcoming age-related challenges in life, and don't let go of the magic!

CHAPTER SEVEN

URINARY TRACT INFECTIONS: MAMA SAID TO DRINK CRANBERRY JUICE . . .

Myths

There are so many myths about urinary tract infections, commonly abbreviated UTIs.

- Myth: To prevent UTIs, clean your vagina with soap and water.
- Myth: If your urine is cloudy or odorous, you have a UTI.
- Myth: Only women can get UTIs.
- Myth: You have to be sexually active to get a UTI.
- Myth: Taking probiotics can protect you from a UTI.
- Myth: For women, wiping from front to back is better than back to front.
- Myth: Drinking cranberry juice or extract can prevent or treat a UTI.

Sorry mama, these are all just myths. This list of myths was compiled by Joanna Langner at Stanford, and given all the myths around UTIs, I thought it was most important to separate truth from fiction.

Defining Urinary Tract Infections

Physicians use the term urinary tract infection to describe an infection of the bladder and urethra, which is the tube that allows urine to flow from the bladder to the world outside of your body. If the infection spreads to the kidneys, it is called pyelonephritis. Symptoms of urinary tract infections include increased urinary frequency, urgency to urinate, burning with urination, blood in the urine, and pain in the mid-lower abdomen above the pubic bone. Sometimes elderly people only experience increased confusion. If the infection spreads to the kidneys, patients experience mid-back discomfort or pain towards one side, often accompanied by fever, shaking chills, and sometimes even nausea and vomiting (see Figure 7.1).

Most UTIs are caused by bacteria that can be found in the gastrointestinal tract, like *Escherichia coli* (*E. coli*). Sexually transmitted infections can also cause infections of the urethra in both men and women.

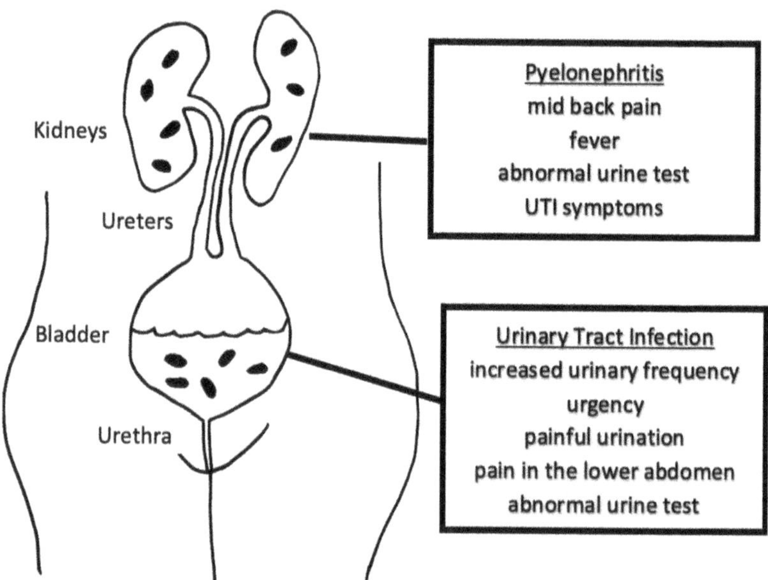

Figure 7.1. Anatomy of urinary tract. This figure also shows the difference between a urinary tract infection and a more serious kidney infection. The black spots are meant to represent clumps of bacteria.

Risk Factors for Urinary Tract Infections

If you have talked with your friends and family, you may have noticed that some people are more likely to get urinary tract infections than others. Here are risk factors that predispose some individuals to UTIs:

- Female Anatomy—Women have shorter urethras than men, making it easier for bacteria to make their way into the bladder. Even among women, the length, width, and angle of the urethra put some women at higher risk for infection than others.
- Sexual Activity—The reason that sex causes UTIs is because the physical act causes bacteria from the genitals and anus to be in direct contact with the urethra. Having a new sex partner and being exposed to new types and strains of bacteria also increase your risk.
- Birth Control—Diaphragms and spermicidal agents can alter anatomy and hold bacteria against the urethra, increasing the risk of infection.
- Menopause—With decreased estrogen, the tissue around the urethra gets dry and shrinks, causing the urethra to widen. This makes it easier for bacteria to climb up the urethra and into the bladder. The absence of estrogen also changes the pH of the vagina, making it harder to ward off bacteria that cause infection.
- Kidney Stones—Stones can trap urine behind the stone like a dam, allowing urine to become stagnant, thereby increasing the risk of UTIs.
- Enlarged Prostate—An enlarged prostate can trap urine in the bladder, also like a dam, allowing urine to become stagnant, thereby increasing the risk of UTIs.
- Prolapsed Bladder—A prolapsed bladder can kink the urethra and create an obstruction causing the same problems as stones and enlarge prostates by blocking urine flow.
- Damaged Nerves, Bladder Weakness, or Surgically Reconstructed Bladder—These can all cause urinary retention that increases the risks of UTIs and may require a patient to put a tube (catheter) in their bladder to drain it several times a day.

- Scarring in the Urethra—Prior infections, such as the sexually transmitted infection gonorrhea, can cause narrowing (strictures) in men's urethra that trap urine in the bladder and increase the risk of UTIs.
- Catheter Use—If a catheter is not inserted using sterile technique, bacteria from the skin can be introduced into the bladder. If the catheter is left in, it provides an open path for the bacteria to enter the bladder. Bacteria are really good at sticking to and climbing the catheter material for easy entry into the bladder.
- Suppressed Immune System—Diseases that impair the immune system, like diabetes or rheumatoid arthritis, or even advanced age, prevent the body from mounting an early defense against the first bacterial invaders, resulting in more frequent infections.
- Recent Urinary Procedure—If procedural equipment is not inserted using sterile technique, bacteria from the skin can be introduced into the bladder. But also, tiny tears in the lining of the urinary tracts from the equipment can also increase the risk of infection.

When to See Your Doctor for a Urinary Tract Infection

If you seldom get urinary tract infections and you have the classic symptoms, then your doctor may be able to prescribe antibiotics by just hearing your story over the phone. However, if you get recurrent infections, or are feeling sick, then you should see your doctor. Your doctor will check your vital signs, feel your abdomen, tap on your kidneys, and, if you are male, check your prostate and epididymis for infection. Then your urine should be tested. Doctors often start with an office dipstick, which will show if your urine has white blood cells, which could indicate infection and nitrites that are produced by bacteria. If those are positive, your doctor may treat you with antibiotics or send your urine for microscopy and culture. Microscopy will provide more specific and accurate information about your urine, such as the exact amount of white blood cells, and the culture will provide information about what type of bacteria is in your urine, how many bacteria are there, and which antibiotics would be best to treat the infection. If the culture suggests a different antibiotic from the one initially prescribed, your doctor will then call you and recommend a change in antibiotics.

Treatment of Urinary Tract Infections

Treatment usually entails a short course of oral antibiotics. Due to increasing antibiotics resistance, on rare occasions, people need to go to the hospital for IV antibiotics to treat a simple urinary tract infection because the bacteria are resistant to all oral antibiotics. If the kidneys are involved, patients often need a brief course of IV antibiotics in the hospital prior to transitioning to oral antibiotics.

Prevention, of course, is always best. I am presenting a range of preventative options that you can discuss with your doctor.

What You Can Do for Yourself

- Drink plenty of water in the range of two to three liters per day. This allows you to flush out bacteria before an infection can take hold.
  - Decrease alcohol and caffeine as they can irritate the bladder.
  - Urinate when you have to. Don't hold urine in your bladder for long periods of time.
  - Empty your bladder as much as possible when urinating. Take your time. Don't rush.
  - Clean the groin (perineal area) once or twice daily with warm water, a mild non-perfumed cleanser, and a sudsy washcloth.
  - Remove garments immediately if they become soiled. Clean the groin (perineal area) twice daily with warm water, cleanser, and washcloth. For individuals who are unable to tell you if they have urinated or had a bowel movement, check incontinence briefs every two hours.
- Women:
  - Urinate after intercourse and after a bowel movement to rinse bacteria from the urethra.

    - Avoid spermicidal jellies and diaphragms (though I'm not sure women use diaphragms anymore!).
    - Avoid douches, sprays, scented powders, and other irritants to the vaginal area.
- Men:
    - Urinate after anal intercourse to rinse bacteria from the urethra.
    - If you are uncircumcised, clear the foreskin daily to avoid bacteria getting trapped near the urethra.
- Some people have bladders that retain urine, and they need to put a tube (catheter) in the urethra to drain urine from the bladder multiple times a day. If you self-catheterize, take extra care to use the sterile technique, and if you have an indwelling catheter, be sure to have it changed monthly. Clean the groin (perineal area) twice daily with warm water, a cleanser, and a washcloth.
- Treat your underlying diseases, such as diabetes, that put you at higher risk of getting more complicated and severe urinary tract infections.

What Your Doctor Can Do

- Confirm the diagnosis and make sure other organs are not infected, like the kidneys or prostate. The doctor can also make sure that an enlarged prostate (see Chapter 10), estrogen deficiency (see Chapter 12), or drooping bladder (see Chapter 9) is not contributing to the infection.
- Your doctor can choose an appropriate antibiotic based on your kidney function, medication allergies, and prior culture results.
- Send your urine off for a culture to ensure that the antibiotics prescribed will work for the bacteria that you have been infected with and check that you don't have a resistant bacterial infection.
- For women, if you have recurrent infections, your doctor can talk to you about prevention methods:

  - If estrogen deficiency is increasing your risk of urinary tract infections, your doctor may prescribe a twice-weekly estrogen cream to your urethra. (More in Chapter 12.)
  - If a dropping bladder (prolapsed bladder) is increasing your risk of urinary tract infections, your doctor may prescribe a pessary. A pessary is a round, relatively flat piece of plastic or silicone that gets placed into the vagina to hold the bladder in place. It fits around the cervix like a diaphragm. If sized and placed correctly, a patient should not be able to feel it. (More in Chapter 9.)
  - Some women need to take antibiotics with intercourse to prevents UTIs.
  - Some women need to take low-dose antibiotics every day, all the time, to prevent UTIs.
- For men, if you have recurrent infections, your doctor can talk to you about prevention methods such as treatment of an enlarged prostate or blockages in the urethra called strictures. (See Chapter 10.)
- Most people get preventative or prophylactic antibiotics around the time of urinary procedures. Ask if they are not offered.
- There are several preventative therapies under investigation. Vaccines and oral medications to stimulate the immune system against the most common bacteria to cause UTIs are under investigation.

Common Patient Stories

At sixty years old, Margaret had four urinary tract infections in one year, and they were more than a nuisance. They were uncomfortable, disrupted her plans for the day, and made her very tired. When she was younger, she remembered having to take nitrofurantoin when she had sex with her husband to prevent urinary tract infections. After he passed away, she hoped that her urinary tract infections were a problem of the past. Unfortunately, now menopause was catching up with her, and the lack of estrogen made her prone to urinary tract infections once again. Reluctant to take medication, it wasn't until the fourth urinary tract infection that she agreed to apply estrogen cream to her urethra twice a week. Margaret now reports that she has only had one urinary tract infection in the past five years, and she has a new beau.

Jim is a sixty-five-year-old gentleman who said that he felt like he was sitting on an uncomfortable rock. It was difficult to describe, but there was an uncomfortable fullness at the base of his penis. He also reported burning when he urinated, having to urinate more frequently, and discomfort in his mid-lower abdomen. From prior exams, I knew that he had an enlarged prostate. At this office visit, his urine test was consistent with a urinary tract infection, and his prostate was very tender. I also learned that he had stopped taking the tamsulosin for his enlarged prostate when the medication ran out, as he just never refilled the prescription. Urine had gotten backed up behind the prostate, became stagnant, and got infected. The infected urine then infected both his bladder and his prostate, which required three weeks of oral antibiotics to treat. Ever since, he has been taking his tamsulosin more reliably and has not had another infection.

More on the Myths

Now, let's delve a bit deeper into the myths.

- Myth: To prevent UTIs, clean your vagina with soap and water.
    - Cleanliness is very important because the groin area is full of bacteria, as described above, but you do not have to apply soap or cleanser up into the vagina. The vagina itself is able to keep itself clean.
- Myth: If your urine is cloudy or odorous, you have a UTI.
    - The odor of urine is stronger with dehydration and can change with foods. It is not a sign of infection. Women often have cloudy urine, and most people with catheters have cloudy urine without having an infection.
- Myth: Only women can get UTIs.
    - Sorry gentleman, you are not immune.
- Myth: You have to be sexually active to get a UTI.
    - Nuns and priests and others who live a celibate life get UTIs.
- Myth: Taking probiotics can protect you from a UTI.

- So far, there isn't any consistent data to support this conclusion. Some have tried D-mannose, vitamin C, as well as probiotics to prevent UTIs. I continue to be frustrated by the lack of data when it comes to supplements for many diseases. This may be because the content within supplements is so highly variable.

- Myth: For women, wiping from front to back is better than back to front.
  - There was a study in women to see if the direction of wiping, front to back or back to front, made a difference. While many still advise wiping from front to back, the study did not find any differences in the frequency of UTIs. I believe the key is to wipe well, making sure you are dry and clean.
- Myth: Drinking cranberry juice or extract can prevent or treat a UTI.
  - I know that some people swear by cranberry juice, while the studies do not show any evidence that it works. My suspicion is that cranberry juice works based on the volume of liquid consumed, just like drinking a lot of water works rather than the properties of the cranberry juice itself. While the cranberry juice and extract do have proanthocyanidins, which block bacteria from sticking to the wall of the bladder, no matter how much you drink, they don't exist in high enough concentrations in the bladder to be effective. The same goes for blueberries. Disappointingly, often, fascinating discoveries in the lab don't pan out in the real world.

Prevention is your best strategy, and there are so many things that can be done to prevent urinary tract infections. Hopefully, you have learned a few new strategies to add to your repertoire. The goal is to avoid the discomfort of urinary tract infections, the side effects of repetitive antibiotic use, and the formation of resistant bacteria that cause urinary tract infections and require complex treatments. Is this possible? Can you reduce the number of urinary tract infections that you have in your lifetime? Absolutely.

CHAPTER EIGHT

URINARY INCONTINENCE: LEAKY PIPES

You Are Not Alone

On a Saturday morning in April, my spouse and I met up with eight of our closest hiking friends and a few ambitious dogs at Echo Lake about seventy-five minutes west and 5,000 feet higher in elevation than the Mile High City where we live. The Chicago Lakes Trail is about eleven miles long, climbing 3,300 feet as it wanders through the Rocky Mountains. Yes, this is how Coloradoans talk about their hikes, with distance, altitude, and ascent included. I'm convinced the intensity qualifies hiking in Colorado as an official sport. The trail connects a series of gorgeous outlooks by way of intermittent, steep, hilly climbs along cliffs, dotted with a few small lakes along the way.

The group was made up of all women, ages forty-four to sixty-five, with, of course, the sixty-five-year-old being the fittest and the fastest. The trail is narrow, and we hike mostly single file. Marcia, our sixty-five-year-old fearless leader, always leads the pack, with her hiking poles available for descents and studded shoe covers dangling from her backpack in anticipation of the icy patches ahead. We like to stay relatively close in case we are to encounter yet another bear, moose, elk, or, what I fear most, mountain lion.

Two miles into the hike, before I even had a chance to notice the first buds of spring, I hear a loud sneeze from someone in the group. I didn't know who, but in my usual style, I commented loudly, "That was a big sneeze." And a voice responded, "And I peed a bit too!"

We were laughing so hard that we had to stop hiking to catch our collective breaths in the thin air. We had all been there at one time or another. How wonderful that I have friends that can talk so freely amongst each other . . . and I'm the only healthcare professional in the group. I know that many people have trouble talking about these topics with their doctor, nonetheless with friends. This was another motivation for me to put these chapters together.

The Definition and Types of Urinary Incontinence

Urinary incontinence or not making it to the toilet in time to urinate is usually no laughing matter. Urinary leakage can come in drips or in floods, and it happens to women and men, though sometimes for different reasons. There are four different types of incontinence (see Figure 8.1):

1. Stress incontinence—due to increased abdominal pressure relative to weak pelvic floor muscles
2. Urge incontinence—due to involuntary contractions of the bladder muscles
3. Overflow incontinence—due to blockage of the urethra, the tube between the bladder and the outside world

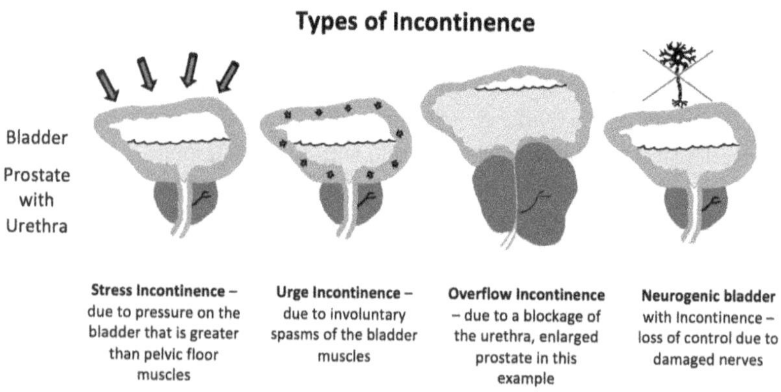

Figure 8.1. Types of incontinence and how they affect your bladder.

4. Neurogenic incontinence—due to impaired functioning of the nerves in the body (nervous system)

Some people have multiple types of urinary incontinence. If the type(s) is not clear, a urologist may recommend urodynamic studies to look at bladder capacity, bladder muscle stability and contractility, and ability to urinate. Let's take a look at them one at a time.

Stress Incontinence

The story described above is the perfect representation of stress incontinence. This is when a sneeze or cough or other cause of increased abdominal pressure overcomes weakened pelvic floor muscles or muscle that holds the urine in (the urethral sphincter) gives way and a few drops of urine leak out. This is much more common in women as they age, especially those who have had multiple childbirths, are obese, and/or menopausal. With menopause, lower estrogen levels lead to lower muscular strength around the urethra and increase the chance of leakage. In men, stress incontinence is most commonly seen after prostate surgery for cancer (a prostatectomy) or a transurethral resection of the prostate (which I rudely call a "rotor rooter") for benign prostatic hyperplasia (BPH) (see Chapter 10).

What You Can Do for Yourself

- Avoid caffeinated beverages, spicy foods, carbonated beverages, alcohol, and citrus, as they irritate the bladder.
- Seek help to quit smoking as smoking irritates the bladder and induces coughing.
- For women with a BMI greater than 25, a 5 percent weight loss can result in a 70 percent improvement in symptoms. Weight loss also helps men but has not been studied as precisely.
- Perform Kegel exercises to strengthen the pelvic floor. Kegel exercises tend to benefit women under sixty years of age the most. However, men and older women do them too for added benefit. Twenty-four contractions (reps) of the urinary sphincter per day are recommended. Kegel exercises can be difficult to do correctly. Consider using a perineometer like the Elvie®

for women, or asking your doctor or a pelvic floor physical therapist if you are doing the exercises correctly.

- Wear incontinence pads. While not a treatment, they can help manage the situation and are recommended over using feminine pads designed for periods (menses). Special pads are also made for men who are averse to wearing larger incontinence briefs.
- Women, ask your doctor if you have a prolapsed bladder and would benefit from a pessary (see Chapter 9). Of note, exercises are more effective than pessaries, but you can also combine the two.

What Your Doctor Can Do

- Help you quit smoking or lose weight.
- Ensure that you are doing Kegel exercises correctly or refer you to a pelvic floor physical therapist.
- Examine you to see if you have a bladder prolapse.
- There are no FDA-approved medications for stress incontinence, though patients on duloxetine (Cymbalta®) demonstrated a 50 percent reduction in incontinence episodes and an improved quality of life. You can consider this option with your doctor.
- When these above options fail, surgery is an alternative for some, while others feel it is not worth the risks and invasion. Your doctor can discuss these options:
  - The surgical procedure of choice for women is the sling operation in which a sling is implanted. The sling implant is a synthetic mesh, piece of your own tissue, or tape that is used to support the urethra. It's like a hammock for your urethra, only not as much fun.
  - In women, an intravesical (in the bladder) balloon device has been shown to improve quality of life and to be safe.
  - Peri/transurethral injections add bulk to the urethra to increase outlet resistance, but the procedure is temporary and works better in people with more stable, immobile urethras (more common in men).

- Implantation of an artificial urinary sphincter is more commonly used in men. It acts like a blood pressure cuff around the urethra that a patient can manually release and refill.
- Men can also undergo a sling procedure, but they are less common.

Future Possibilities

Never give up hope; there are future possibilities being explored every day. Acupuncture has been studied with mixed results, meaning rare studies show benefits, and many do not. Transurethral radiofrequency collagen denaturation has been tried with unknown benefits and also needs further investigation. Pulsed magnetic stimulation is being studied. So far, vaginal laser treatment has yet to show benefit.

Urge Incontinence

This is also sometimes called overactive bladder. Technically, overactive bladder refers to the frequent sensation of needing to urinate. One classic story is of a person who frequently feels like they have to go to the bathroom, especially at night, and then once on the toilet, urinates just a little bit. When a person has an overactive bladder, it becomes urge incontinence as soon as the bladder losses control of urine. This is more common in obese people, people who drink caffeine, and those who tend to be constipated. While this can occur at all ages, it tends to progress with age.

What You Can Do for Yourself

- Avoid caffeinated beverages in particular, though the previously mentioned bladder irritants may also need to be eliminated.
- Weight loss also helps in both men and women but has not been studied as precisely as with stress incontinence.
- Kegel exercises to strengthen the pelvic floor can be helpful, as above with twenty-four contractions (reps) of the urinary sphincter per day. Kegel exercises can be difficult to do

correctly. Consider using a perineometer like the Elvie® for women, or ask your doctor or a pelvic floor physical therapist if you are doing the exercises correctly.

- Treat constipation (see Chapter 11).
- Timed voiding and bladder retraining have been the most successful for my patients.
    - On day one, wake up in the morning, urinate, and record the time. Then record each episode of urination and each episode of incontinence before you go to bed at night.
    - Determine the shortest period of time between urinating and incontinence, and subtract fifteen minutes. Say you urinated at noon and then had an episode of incontinence at 1:15 before you had the urge to go to the bathroom. Your shortest period of time of guaranteed dryness is one hour and fifteen minutes minus fifteen minutes equals one hour.
    - On day two, wake up in the morning, urinate, and record the time. Set an alarm to ring or vibrate every one hour. Every time it rings, get up and try to urinate on the toilet even if you don't have the urge. This will prevent episodes of incontinence.
    - Then, gradually increase the time interval between going to the toilet every few days. Ideally, try to increase the interval between trips to the bathroom by fifteen minutes per day. Your goal is to eventually get to three to four hours.
    - Note it takes at least four to six weeks to see results.

What Your Doctor Can Do

- Help you lose weight.
- Ensure that you are doing Kegel exercises correctly or refer you to a pelvic floor physical therapist.
- Make recommendations to help you treat your constipation.
- Coach you through bladder retraining.
- Discuss medication options, as there are two classes of medications used to treat overactive bladder. Anti-muscarinic medi-

cations like oxybutynin (Ditropan®) and tolterodine (Detrol®) are the most frequently used but have a lot of side effects that I don't particularly like for older patients, such as dizziness, drowsiness, and blurry vision. The newest class of medication is a B3 adrenergic receptor agonist, mirabegron (Myrbetriq®). It has fewer side effects and is my preferred medication treatment, but it may be more expensive for patients depending on their insurance.

- Review procedures to help with urge incontinence, such as botulinum toxin A injections (Botox®) that last about nine months.

Future Possibilities

On the horizon, you are soon to see new treatments. Treatment using electrical stimulation is still being actively explored. Percutaneous stimulation of the tibial nerve (PTNS) is being utilized with anecdotal improvements. Sacral neuromodulation has shown more consistent improvement but involves surgical implantation of a stimulation device. Hypnotherapy was studied and was not as effective as medication. Unfortunately, acupuncture reported conflicting results again.

Overflow Incontinence

Overflow incontinence is like having a dam in a river that just can't hold back the tide and water starts to flow over the dam and leaks out. Most people with overflow incontinence are not able to fully empty their bladder when they urinate. They often start and stop their urine stream trying to empty the bladder. After urinating, the partially emptied bladder is quick to fill up again and overflow the dam. Sometimes, the dam is the prostate, a urethral stricture in men (scar tissue kinking or blocking the urethra), bladder stones, or weak bladder muscles. Either way, the leakage of urine is often sudden, unexpected, and of larger volume. It can even occur at night.

What You Can Do for Yourself

- For women, medications rarely treat overflow incontinence. Intermittent self-catheterization in which a person inserts a tube through the urethra into the bladder four times a day may be necessary to empty the bladder. Some women opt for a continuous indwelling Foley catheter to drain urine, but that puts a person at much higher risk for recurrent urinary tract infections. When possible, intermittent self-catheterization is preferred.

What Your Doctor Can Do

- Teach you how to properly use a catheter
- Sometimes, surgery can help correct overflow incontinence by removing stones or abnormal growths obstructing the flow of urine
- In men, overflow incontinence is usually caused by an enlarged prostate. Medications can be used to shrink the prostate, helping the bladder to empty more completely with urination and improve urinary flow (see Chapter 10).
- Men can also benefit from surgery to remove tissue from the prostate that is obstructing the urethra. The most common procedure is the transurethral resection of the prostate (TURP) (see Chapter 10).
- Of note, post-urination dribbling of a few drops in men is rarely dangerous or from a disease

Neurogenic Bladder

People whose nerves to their bladder have been damaged can experience incontinence. This is commonly seen in diseases such as multiple sclerosis, Parkinson's, spinal cord injuries, and diabetes mellitus. This occurs because patients either can't feel when their bladder is full and don't know when to empty it, or they have lost control of the muscles that allow them to hold and release urine voluntarily. The most common symptom is being unable to control urination; some also report a weak stream, frequent urination, and urgency to get to the toilet when they need to go.

What You Can Do for Yourself

- Avoid caffeinated beverages in particular, though the previously mentioned bladder irritants may also need to be eliminated.
- Weight loss also helps in both men and women but has not been studied as precisely as with stress incontinence.
- Some people need to perform intermittent self-catheterization in which a person inserts a tube through the urethra into the bladder four times a day in order to empty the bladder. Some people opt for a continuous indwelling Foley catheter to drain urine, but that puts a person at much higher risk for recurrent urinary tract infections. When possible, intermittent self-catheterization is preferred.

What Your Doctor Can Do

- Help you lose weight
- Teach you how to properly use a catheter
- If the bladder is overactive, the same medications for urge incontinence can be used. As mentioned, there are two classes of medications used to treat overactive bladder. Anti-muscarinic medications like oxybutynin (Ditropan®) and tolterodine (Detrol®) are the most frequently used but have a lot of side effects. The newest class of medication, a B3 adrenergic receptor agonist, mirabegron (Myrbetriq®), has fewer side effects, but I have found it to be more expensive for my patients.
- Doctors can perform procedures to help with neurogenic bladders, including botulinum toxin A injections (Botox®), which last about nine months, bladder augmentation, and creating ileal conduits. Bladder augmentation is a surgery that removes a piece of your sigmoid colon (large intestine) and adds it to your bladder to make it bigger. An ileal conduit surgery creates a new bladder from your small intestine, and the urine

collects in this new bladder and then empties into a bag that is attached to the outside of your body like a colostomy bag.

- Sacral neuromodulation has shown more consistent improvement but involves surgical implantation of a stimulation device.

Incontinence and Dementia

People with dementia also struggle with incontinence. Sometimes, they have one of the conditions that we mentioned above. When there is not a problem with the bladder or urinary tract, people with dementia can remain continent for a long time if taken to the toilet every two hours during the day, easing strain on caregivers. Dementia robs people of the ability to recognize that their bladder is full, the ability to remember how to ask for assistance, and to find the bathroom, but people remember what to do on the toilet well into the severe stages of dementia. Scheduled toileting is the best way to manage incontinence with people who have dementia. Set a timer.

Facing a New Reality

I have a close family member who underwent a prostatectomy for prostate cancer and experienced a very unpleasant but relatively common side effect. After surgery, he was left with continuous stress incontinence throughout the day. If any pressure is placed on his bladder from internal organs or muscles from the abdomen, the urinary sphincter that once held back urine is so weak that it is overcome by spurts of urine. He leaks at least half of his daily volume of urine just walking around doing his routine activities. Imagine sitting on the couch watching a movie and realizing that you have to urinate. Then in the ten steps it takes to get to the bathroom, your abdominal muscles put enough pressure on your bladder to gradually empty it before you even make it to the bathroom door.

The solution has been male incontinence pads that are slightly larger than feminine hygiene products that fit over the penis and absorb urine. They prevent leaks and keep the skin dry and rash-free, but they are a nuisance. They are expensive, embarrassing to buy, difficult to discreetly dispose of in a men's bathroom, hot to wear, get heavy when wet, and need to be on hand at all times.

Sometimes as we age, we can prevent unpleasant changes. Sometimes, we get things that are treatable. And other times, we need to let ourselves grieve for what is lost, get angry at our new circumstances, and then learn to adapt and reframe the way we view our lives. I watched him go through these stages. It is not that he still doesn't get frustrated from time to time, but he recognized that he is still alive and that the cancer didn't take his life. He feels otherwise well, is in good physical shape, and can do all of the things he had done before the surgery. He has also helped shepherd other men who have struggled with a new diagnosis of prostate cancer, having to choose among several treatment options and learning to live with the outcomes.

On the other hand, I have had quite a few patients lose ten pounds and come dancing into my office because their incontinence is gone. Like anything that affects the body, symptoms can be mild, moderate, or severe. No matter which, there are so many ways to improve one's situation and recapture elements of your life you think you may have lost.

CHAPTER NINE
PROLAPSES: OOPS, I THINK SOMETHING FELL OUT

When the Patient Is Right

Recently, a female patient came to the office wearing tight jeans and tried to walk into the office with her legs crossed. She was horrified as most would be of the idea, let alone the sensation, that something was falling out of her. "Oops, I think something fell out!" she exclaimed in horror. She was correct. In her case, her uterus had fallen and was starting to hang outside of her body. The diagnosis was a prolapsed uterus. With minimal effort, I was able to put it back in its proper place, but the fix was only temporary. She uttered, "I've never heard of this before!" It is fairly common for women to prolapse their uterus, bladder, or rectum. The reason she had never heard about it is that there are some diagnoses that people don't like to talk about. Good thing for you, doctors are willing to talk about anything and everything.

This chapter may make some folks blush, but it is important to read and to learn about prolapses for the women in our community and for the women in your lives that we love.

Definition of Pelvic Organ Prolapse

Pelvic organ prolapse is a common problem that occurs as women age and the muscles and ligaments around the uterus and bladder stretch and become weakened. Prolapse means the descending or dropping of an organ.

Because of a stretched-out and weakened pelvis, the uterus, the bladder, and the rectum drop from their usual positions. The diagram in Figure 9.1 shows a cross section of normal anatomy in the upper left-hand corner. As those ligaments and muscles loosen, either the bladder, uterus, or rectum can droop or prolapse following the path of gravity, rearranging the normal anatomy. The uterus and bladder can fall so far that they come out of the body entirely. (If you enjoyed the game "guess how this picture is different from the first . . ." it might make this figure a bit less horrifying and perhaps a little fun?)

Pelvic organ prolapse is more common among women who have had multiple pregnancies or if other family members have had prolapses. Other risk factors include babies greater than nine pounds at birth, obesity, chronic constipation, chronic coughing, and/or straining. Prolapses can be mild to severe, and symptoms range from no symptoms at all to having your internal part dangling between your legs.

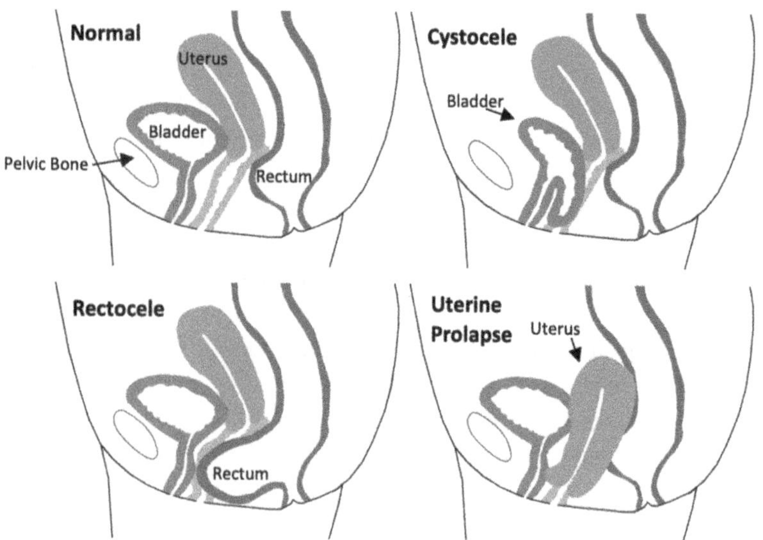

Figure 9.1. A comparison of normal female anatomy and different types of prolapse. Bladder prolapses are called cystoceles and rectal prolapses are called rectoceles. Uterine prolapses do not have a confusing medical name.

What You Can Do for Yourself

- Go to your doctor if you notice a feeling of heaviness in the pelvis, pain with intercourse, a bulge in the vaginal opening, are unable to empty your bladder completely, have constipation, and/or have frequent bladder infections.
- See if you can tell if the symptoms worsen with standing or walking for long periods of time, as gravity makes the prolapse worse.
- Tell your doctor what you think might be happening or what you are worried about. Explain your symptoms even if the doctor doesn't ask.
- Don't wait. The problem is easier to fix if you seek help early.

What Your Doctor Can Do

- The diagnosis can be made by a pelvic exam and may require a rectal exam looking for bulges in the vaginal canal caused by a misplaced uterus, bladder, or rectum.
- Your doctor can review non-surgical or surgical treatments:
    - The non-surgical option entails the placement of a removable pessary. A pessary is a round, flat, flexible silicone or plastic device that is inserted into the vagina and goes around the cervix like a diaphragm. It holds the uterus and bladder in place, providing mechanical support so that they cannot drop from their normal position. (See Figure 9.2.) Pessaries need to be removed and cleaned every three months by the patient or their doctor to avoid bacteria buildup and odor.
    - If prolapse is more severe, surgical prolapse repair, with or without a hysterectomy, is recommended. This surgery can be done through the vagina most of the time with limited incisions and a faster recovery.

Older patients with pessaries typically come to my office every three months so that I can take them out, clean them, and put them back in. For some, pessaries can be difficult to reach and reposition when replaced. It

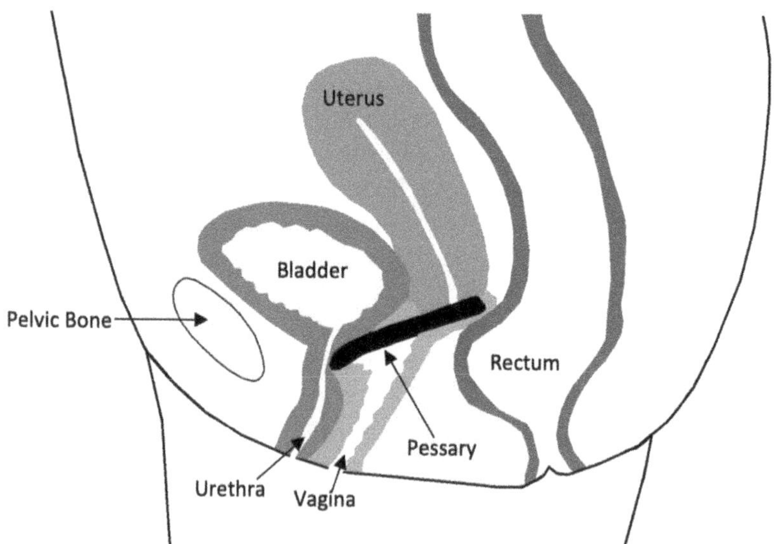

Figure 9.2. Female anatomy demonstrating the placement of a pessary.

is easy and quick for a doctor to do, and patients seem to tolerate it well. Most say that it is much easier than a speculum exam and pap smear and easier for me to do it than for them to try to do it themselves. It also gives me an excuse to check in and catch-up with my patients at least every three months.

Team Approach

Nobody is good at everything. I have gone to formal schooling for twenty-four years, practiced medicine for decades, and am reading continuously. Yet, I still call on peers and specialists with medical questions every week. That is how I help my patients and how I keep learning. As you can hopefully tell, I love to recant stories and to translate what I know about medicine from medical jargon to a language everyone can understand. While my spelling is pretty good, my grammar needs some help. Ask any of my patients who are English teachers and who dutifully read my weekly newsletters. For help, I call upon copy editors. As I embarked on writing this book, I employed different editors to help me ensure that my ideas were well developed and flowed coherently, a book agent to help me find a publisher, another copy editor to proof and set the pages, illustrators, a publisher, etc. Finding success often requires me to identify when I need help and to select the right team of experts to assist me.

Sometimes you can take on the aging process yourself, doing what you can, with full self-reliance. Other times, you must employ the help of others. If you think you have a prolapse, this is just one example of a time when the best thing you can do to help yourself is to ask for assistance. There are doctors out there qualified, willing, and able to make your life better. Don't pass them by. Seek out help along your journey so that you can age like a fine bottle of wine and not an expired jug of grape juice!

CHAPTER TEN
BENIGN PROSTATIC HYPERPLASIA: BEDTIME PEEING HOTSHOT

What Is a Prostate?

Unfortunately, BPH does not stand for "bedtime peeing hotshot." Although, now that you think of it, if you are male, you probably do get up to pee at night more than anyone else in your household. Why not accept a title for that? It is a hard-earned reward given the many nights of disturbed sleep you have endured, followed only by the struggle of endless days with drooping eyelids. Too bad having a big prostate is nothing to brag about.

The prostate is an organ reserved strictly for males. It produces some of the fluid that makes up semen, and its muscles are responsible for the forceful release of semen during ejaculation. It is important for men to know where their prostate is (see Figure 10.1). Occasionally, a male will come into the office and identify discomfort in the prostate. This is often related to a prostate infection (prostatitis). The prostate is located under the bladder, and the urethra passes through the prostate, carrying urine from the bladder through the prostate and through the penis to the outside environment. You will see from the diagram that the prostate is located at the base of the penis, with just a bit of pelvic floor muscle separating the prostate from the base of the penial shaft.

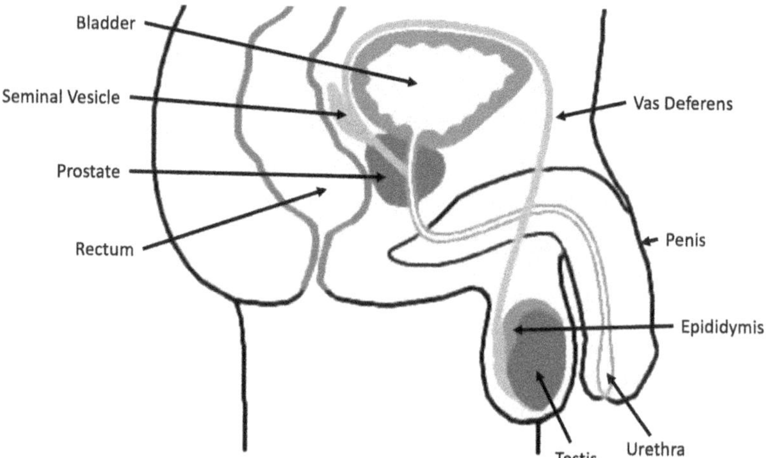

Figure 10.1. Anatomy of the male. Note the prostate deep in the male pelvis.

Defining Benign Prostatic Hyperplasia

BPH stands for benign prostatic hyperplasia. Starting around age forty, the prostate enlarges on average 1.6 percent per year. The cause is unknown, but we do know that young men who lose their testicles early due to testicular cancer do not get BPH. Testosterone is the leading suspect being investigated. Some people will also develop nodules in their prostate from BPH, and other times, these nodules may be indicative of cancer.

Only 25 percent of men will develop symptoms that require treatment. In the second diagram, you can see that as the prostate enlarges, it narrows the urethra, causing a partial blockage of the tube that lets urine escape from the body. It also presses against the muscles at the outlet of the bladder, causing the bladder muscles to become weakened. As the bladder distends with urine when you need the muscles to be at their strongest, the muscles get even weaker (see Figure 10.2).

Men with the largest prostates develop a weak, slow urinary stream, hesitancy of urination, straining to initiate and maintain urination, and prolonged urination. Multiple trips to the bathroom at night are common (nocturia). Often, there is an uncontrollable urge to go, but only a small

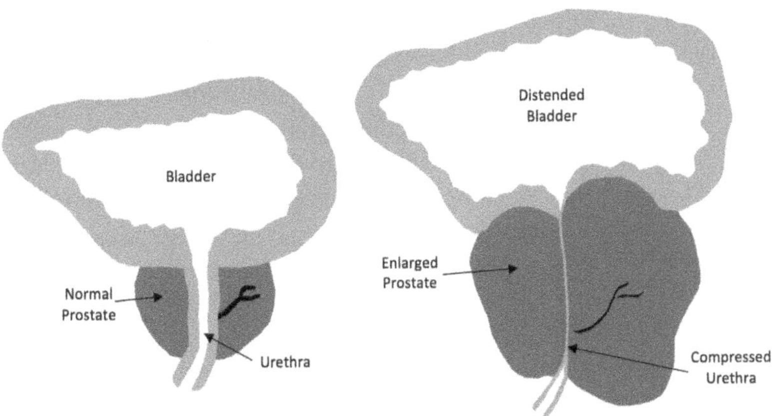

Figure 10.2. A comparison of normal anatomy with how an enlarged prostate affects the bladder and urethra.

amount of urine is produced. Where is the good news, you ask? BPH does not increase your risk of prostate cancer.

When to See Your Doctor

If you have symptoms of BPH, you should see your doctor. After your doctor collects an extensive history, the physical will include an examination of the abdomen, pelvis, and perineum, a motor and sensory exam of the pelvis and lower extremities, and a digital rectal exam. Yes, a digital rectal exam is necessary to assess for tenderness and bogginess that may indicate infection, asymmetry, or nodules that raise suspicion for prostate cancer and assess the strength of the anal muscle (sphincter) and sensation in the perineum. You are permitted to whine when your doctor says it is time to do a rectal exam, as you won't be the first. In fact, it is the most common reaction when I say it's time to examine your prostate: "Really, do we have to?" While laboratory tests like the PSA are helpful to assess prostate volume, they still miss 20 to 30 percent of prostate cancers. My advice to you is to let your doctor do the prostate exam.

Your doctor may also ask you to urinate and use an ultrasound on your lower abdomen to measure how much urine is still left in your bladder. This will determine how much urine you retain after emptying your bladder. Most men have less than 35mL in their bladders after urination, but doctors tend to become concerned when that number exceeds 250 to 300mL. Urodynamic studies, which assess bladder capacity, bladder muscle stability, and contractility and ability to urinate, may also be ordered by your physician if they think it will change their management of your symptoms.

Many patients ask me when they should begin treatment for their BPH. That decision is entirely up to you. Some patients elect to treat their symptoms so that they can get a more continuous night's rest without having to get up and go to the bathroom. Others start developing urinary tract infections or anxiety over not being able to empty their bladders. Symptoms and the patient's desire to have those symptoms mitigated determine when to begin treatment.

What You Can Do for Yourself

- Reduce fluid intake after dinner.
- Limit alcohol, caffeine, spicy food, citrus, and anything that can irritate the bladder.
- Treat constipation (see Chapter 11).
- Eat a diet rich in sesame seeds, salmon, bell peppers, tomatoes, avocados, green leafy vegetables, and tofu. The degree of benefit is unknown, but for most people, it can't hurt.
- Increase activity, including regular strenuous exercise.
- Maintain normal body weight.
- Kegel exercises to strengthen the pelvic floor can help. Twenty-four contractions (reps) of the urinary sphincter and the muscles that prevent you from passing gas per day are recommended. Your spouse just might thank me!
- Some patients benefit from timed voiding, where they go to the bathroom to urinate every two hours while awake rather than when they feel like they have to go.
- Other patients find it helpful to "double-void," where after urinating, they wait a minute and try to go again, before leaving the bathroom.
- Avoid diphenhydramine (Benadryl®), pseudoephedrine (Sudafed®), and other decongestants. Try guaifenesin (Mucinex®) and nasal sprays instead if you have a cold. Try loratadine (Claritin®), cetirizine (Zyrtec®), or fexofenadine (Allegra®)

without the "D" for allergies. These last three medications have some effect on urination but much less.

- If you are on a water pill (diuretic), like Lasix®, ask your doctor when in the day you should take them to avoid having to urinate at night.
- Never pass up the chance to use a bathroom.
- If traveling, request an aisle seat.
- Know where bathrooms are located.
- Make your night trips to the bathroom safe by having a night-light and ensure a clear path to the bathroom.
- Over-the-counter treatments—With saw palmetto, some patients report improvement in urinary flow and decreased urination at night. The CVS brand has worked well for some of my patients with early BPH. South African star grass (*Hypoxis rooperi*) and African plum (*Pygeum africanum*) have been used by patients who report improved urine flow and fewer symptoms. Stinging nettle and ryegrass pollen have been advertised to help with the prostate, but I have not seen or heard of any data or stories. Because the long-term safety and efficacy of over-the-counter products are not known, the American Urologic Association recommends against them. Some of the combination formulas for the prostate contain nonsteroidal anti-inflammatory medications (NSAIDs) that can affect the heart, stomach, and kidneys, so be sure to bring the bottles of anything you take to your doctor.

What Your Doctor Can Do

- Help you reduce alcohol intake.
- Provide tips on treating constipation (see Chapter 11).
- Encourage exercise and weight loss.
- Ensure that you are doing Kegel exercises correctly or refer you to a pelvic floor physical therapist.
- Review medication options:
    - Alpha blockers, like tamsulosin (Flomax®), alfuzosin (Uroxatral®), terazosin (Hytrin®), doxazosin (Cardura®), silodosin (Rapaflo®), and prazosin (Minipress®), relax the

smooth muscles of the prostate and bladder, allowing urine to flow more freely after about seven days of use. This is the preferred first-line medication for the treatment of BPH.
  - 5-Alpha Reductase inhibitors such as finasteride (Proscar®) and dutasteride (Avodart®) prevent progression of BPH and help shrink the prostate by 25 percent in twelve to eighteen months. The effects start to become apparent around six to eight weeks, and symptoms continue to improve for over a year.
  - Phosphodiesterase 5 inhibitors like tadalafil (Cialis®) relax the smooth muscle in the bladder and prostate, and patients report improved symptoms.
- Determine if you have bladder problems as well; they may need to be treated separately (see Chapter 8).
- Surgical options are considered when symptoms are moderate to severe and are not improved with medical therapy. If you are still experiencing unremitting symptoms, urinary retention in the bladder or kidneys, recurrent urinary tract infections, visible blood in the urine, or recurrent bladder stones, you likely need surgery. There are many, many different types of surgery, and the type of surgery your doctor will recommend is determined by the size and shape of the prostate, your bleeding risk, presence of stones, symptoms, and sexual function, and desire for its preservation. Here's the current overwhelming list of options you may hear about:
  - Minimally invasive surgical treatments include water vapor thermal therapy and prostatic urethral lift
  - Prostatic ablative therapies include transurethral resection of the prostate (most common), transurethral vaporization of the prostate, transurethral incision of the prostate, photoselective vaporization of the prostate, laser enucleation of the prostate, robot-assisted waterjet ablation of the prostate, transurethral microwave therapy, and simple prostatectomy
- Investigational/emerging technologies include prostatic arterial embolization.

Research Online

I know that some of you will go online and research each and every one of the procedures that I just listed. I think that it is a great idea to learn as much as you can so that you can approach your doctor as an informed partner. Remember, the Internet is full of dangerous information and not just about medicine. When you read something, consider the source. Is it coming from a physician? Good information comes from non–medical doctors, too, but it can be difficult to assess credibility without at least the validation of a medical degree. Is it just one, or do multiple doctors at different practice sites provide similar information? If it is just one, watch out for scams or other motivations for secondary gain. The Urology Care Foundation has a lot of great information for patients and is endorsed by the American Urological Association.

Take what you have learned and work with your physician. Why do physicians need an additional seven-plus years of medical education after college? They need to understand the science of the body. They will be familiar with diagnostic options and treatment algorithms *and* the science behind them. This allows physicians to individualize diagnostic and treatment plans specifically for you and your symptoms.

Learning to Trust My Patients

When I was a young medical student and older men denied symptoms of BPH, I assumed they were lying and that they just didn't want to tell a young lady. I have since learned many things. First, trust your patients. I really did think this was a universal process of aging until residency, when I learned that only 25 percent of men are afflicted. However, 25 percent is still a lot of men. Some of my patients get up three to four times a night before they seek any help. My heart breaks for them. Such sleep disruptions every night sounds absolutely miserable and will lead to weight gain and health decline that will only worsen symptoms, creating a downward spiral.

There are many features of aging that can become a downward spiral if you give up and accept them as inevitable, but I won't let you do that until you are at least one hundred. Why? Because my one-hundred-plus patients have never given up, and that is why they are over one hundred. They have never just accepted their numeric fate. They learned to work with the strengths they had and to build the life they wanted for themselves. This is a treatable problem. Again, you just have to take the appropriate steps and work with your doctor to get on top of the problem! As I said to the women in the last chapter, seek out help along your journey so that you can age like a fine bottle of wine and not an expired jug of grape juice!

CHAPTER ELEVEN
CONSTIPATION: CONSTIPATION MAKES ME WAIT

An Everyday Worry

Want to hear a poop joke? Never mind, they always stink. I have a lot of patients who spend their entire days perseverating over whether or not they will have a bowel movement that day or the next. But I never question their concern and always listen carefully to the wisdom of my elders. Perhaps in a few years, that will be me—sitting on the sofa with my dogs and cats in front of the crackling fireplace drinking my laxative tea with a fiber supplement mixed in, munching on fiber crackers!

This is a real problem for patients as they age. Without daily bowel movements, patients experience abdominal pain, bloating, rectal pain, bleeding, loss of appetite, nausea, and even vomiting. There are several reasons why constipation is more common among older individuals.

Understanding Constipation

Constipation occurs when bowel movements become firmer, less frequent, and more difficult to pass. Constipation can be defined as having less than three bowel movements per week. However, if those bowel movements aren't large enough to evacuate the contents of your bowels, your intestines might still be full of stool. Bowels require several things to move smoothly: that you drink plenty of fluids, get regular exercise so that your abdominal muscles can help stimulate your intestines to push stool forward, and eat plenty of fiber.

Think about what happens to people over time. Older people tend to drink fewer fluids, become more dehydrated, move less, and tend to eat less food in general, including fiber. The main job of the large intestine, also called the colon, is to absorb water out of your stool. The longer the stool stays in the large intestine before you have a bowel movement, the more water that is reabsorbed from the stool, and the harder it becomes. This is why when you are very constipated, you feel like you are trying to pass cement or small rocks. You should not go more than forty-eight hours without passing stool because all the water is drawn out and the hard stool can give you bleeding hemorrhoids, cause tearing when the large pieces come out (fissures), get stuck in the rectum (obstruction), and cause rectal tissue to push out of your body (prolapse). Think of your intestines as a long plumbing pipe. If it gets clogged with stool, it will back up just like a sink, causing food and liquid to move in the opposite direction. When this occurs, it causes nausea and vomiting, painful bloating, and abdominal cramps.

What You Can Do for Yourself

- Drink at least six full glasses of water per day in addition to other beverages, unless you have been told by your doctor to restrict fluid intake.
- Add fiber to your diet. You can do this with prunes, prune juice, bran cereal, pumpkin, or other fruit and vegetables. Some people prefer to take a fiber supplement like Benefiber®, Citrucel®, or Metamucil®. I find that Benefiber® is the least gassy, but everyone's intestines are different.
    - Unfortunately, fiber alone is not enough to overcome constipation caused by narcotic pain medication.
- Exercise most days of the week to stimulate your intestines.
- Don't ignore the urge to have a bowel movement. If you have to go, use the bathroom, even if you are at the grocery store.
- Some people use stool softeners like docusate (Colace®), but the data suggests that they are minimally helpful, if at all.
- Some laxatives draw water into the intestines to soften and flush stool, such as polyethylene glycol (MiraLAX®), lactulose, and magnesium citrate. Do not use magnesium-based products if you have problems with your kidney function.

- Laxatives that stimulate the muscles to move stool forward include bisacodyl and senna. I'm a big fan of senna tea (e.g., Smooth Move®), as you can titrate the dose based on the length of time you brew the tea. I also find that the warm water stimulates the bowels and that the combination can be less explosive than the pills.
- Lubricant laxatives like glycerin suppositories can help get the bowels moving. It can be helpful to alternate oral and rectal treatments for constipation when it is severe to avoid too much bloating and nausea.
- Enemas can also be very effective if a patient is able to hold them. As patients age, I find that they are less able to hold them for the required amount of time. Be careful to read the packaging on the enema boxes. Those with magnesium are not appropriate for patients with kidney problems.
- I do not recommend drinking mineral oil. Too many patients have swallowed the medicine incorrectly and ended up with this oily substance in their lungs with no way to remove it.
- Acupuncture was shown to be helpful in one short-term study.
- Some people inappropriately contract the pelvic floor muscles and the muscle that lets the stool out (external anal sphincter) when defecating. Pelvic floor physical therapy and electromyography feedback can help patients who have muscle dysfunction.
- Surgery is available to repair rectoceles, where the rectum bulges into the vagina, making it more difficult to naturally aim the stool towards the exit opening (anus) (see Figure 9.1). Some women with rectoceles find it easier to have a bowel movement when they are wearing a tampon, place a finger in the vagina, or put some pressure on the skin between the vagina and the rectum to reduce the bulge.

What Your Doctor Can Do

- Let you know if it is safe to take laxatives with magnesium.
- Help you come up with a bowel regimen from all of the available options.

- Prescription medications are also available when over-the-counter medications fail to work.
    - Prescription medications include non-digestible sugars like lactulose that draw water into the intestines to help soften stool. As the water enters the intestines, the intestines stretch, causing some cramping but also stimulating the bowels to squeeze the stool and move it forward (peristalsis). Lubiprostone (Amitiza®), linaclotide (Linzess®), and placanatide (Trulance®) are newer medications for irritable bowel syndrome (IBS) with constipation that I see being used for elderly people with chronic constipation with success. Colchicine and misoprostol with polyethylene glycol have also been used but are not preferred due to risks and side effects. These medications are not generally recommended for chronic use.
- If you have developed a prolapse or rectocele, you may benefit from surgery. Your doctor can examine you and make recommendations for treatment.

Drinking Enough Water

Many patients find it difficult to drink enough water. Can you find a creative way to track your hydration? Many hospitals give out two-liter water jugs that have incremental marks that let you know how much water you have drunk that day. They are heavy and likely remind you of days you would rather forget. Do you have a favorite glass? Treat yourself to a new mug with a picture or saying that makes you happy. Perhaps have one made with a picture of your family or pets. How much water does it hold? How many cupfuls do you need to drink to equal sixty-four ounces? If that seems like too much, start with forty-eight ounces.

If your favorite cup is twenty ounces, can you drink three cupfuls a day? Make it your own personal experiment. Do it for two weeks. At the end of two weeks, do you look or feel any differently?

Anabelle got a pink cup with a picture of her cat to help motivate her to drink more water. For her, taking MiraLAX® every other day solved her problems with constipation. Joan chose a cup with a picture of her seven grandchildren and found a cup of Smooth Move® Tea every evening kept her regular. Dan couldn't drink a lot of water because of his heart failure, so he took two Senna® pills every night before bed. Elizabeth tried drinking more water from her cup from her favorite travel destination, adding fiber to her diet, exercising daily, and taking MiraLAX® with two Senna® pills every morning and night. Despite all of that, she had minimal relief. After talking to her doctor, lactulose was added to her regimen. Despite its shockingly sweet taste, she is happy to be having bowel movements daily!

When to Call Your Doctor

If constipation is new for you, is associated with blood in your stools, severe pain, weight loss, or you have not had a bowel movement in four to five days, call your physician. When these methods listed above don't work, a patient may require disimpaction where a doctor or nurse has to physically remove the stool from the rectum. Of note, if you are constipated, it often takes ten to twelve bowel movements to empty your bowels. One good bowel movement is usually not enough. So, if you have only had one small movement, you should still call your doctor.

Constipation Is Serious Business

As people reach the old-old stage of their life, anything that disrupts their equilibrium can cause confusion, and then the family and doctors begin a hunt trying to determine the cause of the confusion. The most common winner on the racetrack of possibilities is a urinary tract infection, but close at its heels is constipation. When I worked at the hospital, patients would come to the emergency room too confused to tell us what was wrong and, after a thorough exam, reveals a distended gas- and stool-filled abdomen. We would provide the miracle treatment—a bowel regimen! We would place orders so that nurses could give fluids, laxatives, and an enema. The magic would happen, and they would leave a few hours later as if nothing were amiss, confusion gone, back to their usual selves.

One woman had such bad constipation that she needed to be kept overnight to allow her bowels to empty. She was discharged home with home health services feeling great. Five days later, she returned to the hospital, only this time with dehydration from too much diarrhea. She was very afraid of getting constipated again, and she was a bit forgetful. She admittedly couldn't remember if she had had a bowel movement each day or if she had taken a laxative, so she kept taking laxatives. The easy solution for her was to make a "Poop Chart" for the bathroom that would help her remember if she had gone that day, and if she missed a day, then she would take her laxatives. Problem solved!

This is another area of personal care where preventative care goes a long way to avoid discomfort and frequent encounters with the healthcare system. While I list solutions for managing constipation, sometimes you have to think a bit outside the box to ensure that the tips work for you. By creating a chart, this patient and I thought outside the box to help to avoid return trips to the hospital. How can you find ways to incorporate the tips that are the most important for you into your life so that you can get on with life and not have to worry about your bowels?

CHAPTER TWELVE
SEXUAL DYSFUNCTION: THE SPARK CAN'T LIGHT THE FIRE

It Is Natural and Normal

There are very romantic mating stories in nature. The albatrosses are migratory birds that can spend years at sea without landing. When they do come home to the Galapagos Islands for mating, they always come back to their lifelong partners. Humpback whales sing songs to their mates. Some species like the sage grouse dance to attract their mate. Adelie penguins are said to gift their female mates with smooth, shiny pebbles.

Others are less romantic and more sexual. Bonobo apes have quite the reputation in the wild for their promiscuity. They engage in a wide variety of sexual acts for reproduction, recreation, to make friends, form group bonds, and as currency. They enjoy sex with both sexes and aren't particularly jealous. Interestingly, they are one of the few non-human animals to have sex face-to-face.

As varied as sexual practices are in the wild, so are the sexual practices of humans. Regardless of whether a person identifies as heterosexual, homosexual, bisexual, or pansexual (not limited in affection by sex or gender identity), one thing is inevitable. The way an individual experiences sex and sexual intimacy changes over a lifetime. Because this is a book about aging, we are going to focus on this segment of sexual life.

Some people continue to have a very active sex life throughout their golden years, and others do not. There is no right or wrong number of times that one should have sex. Likewise, there are no rules about who one should have sex with or how, as long as it is between consenting adults. It is most important that each participating individual is enjoying the experience, is doing what is comfortable for them, and that *no one* should ever be forced to have sex when they don't want to.

Sexual Challenges in Men

Males first. Most importantly, don't hesitate to talk to your doctor about these issues. They are very common. Among forty-year-old men, 40 percent acknowledge impaired sexual function. Among fifty-year-old men, 50 percent acknowledge impaired sexual function. Among sixty-year-old men, 60 percent acknowledge impaired sexual function . . . and the trend continues. Men in good health are more likely to be sexually active as they age. Compared to women, men lose more years of sexually active life due to poor health. (Perhaps that is good motivation to exercise and eat healthier!) Men tend to hold on to their libido longer than their function, further magnifying the frustration posed by issues of erectile dysfunction and abnormal ejaculation. They also notice that their erections take longer to build and are not as firm. Orgasms have diminished intensity and duration, and semen now dribbles rather than explodes. Proper function requires healthy and intact vascular, neurologic, hormonal, and psychological systems. While men can have orgasms and ejaculate without an erection, they often find the experience less satisfying.

Decreased Libido

Some men experience a decrease in libido. The word libido refers to sexual desire. There are numerous causes, and often, men with decreased libido are struggling for multiple reasons for their lost or dwindling libido. If you struggle with decreased libido, take a look at the following list to see if any of these may be making your problems worse:

- Medications—some antidepressants, narcotic pain medicine, some medications for benign prostatic hyperplasia; if you think any of these might be the cause, don't just stop them, talk with your doctor first.
- Alcohol

- Depression
- Fatigue
- Recreational drugs—with the legalization of marijuana in my state, I see this with much greater frequency.
- Relationship problems
- Other medical diseases
- Testosterone deficiency—although most men think this is the problem and the easy fix, it usually isn't.

Erectile Dysfunction

When it comes to erectile dysfunction (ED), exercise reduces your risk, while obesity, smoking, having a sedentary lifestyle, and having multiple medical problems increase your risk. If you have diabetes, heart disease, high blood pressure, high cholesterol, or obstructive sleep apnea, work with your doctor to make sure that these are optimally managed to prevent damage to the blood vessels and nerves that supply the penis. Of note, weight loss and increased physical activity improved ED in one-third of patients. Medications such as antidepressants and some diuretics can affect erectile function. In addition to reviewing your medication, your doctor should also check your thyroid function, as both hypo- and hyperthyroid can affect sexual function.

We know that men with low testosterone levels (<225ng/dL) struggle with low libido and erectile dysfunction. We also know that men who take testosterone and medications for erectile dysfunction are more likely to get nocturnal erections. Unfortunately, there is no consistent data to show that the combination or testosterone alone results in the return of erectile function for sexual activity.

Ejaculatory Disorders

A smaller number of aging males experience ejaculatory disorders. These include ejaculating within one minute of penetration or intense sexual activity (premature ejaculation), ejaculation occurring later than one desires (delayed ejaculation), inability to ejaculate (anejaculation), releasing semen into the bladder with orgasm only to be expelled later with urination (retrograde ejaculation), and the inability to achieve an orgasm (anorgasmia).

Often, multiple causes contribute to these conditions. Your doctor will review your medications, recreational drug use, any nerve problems, surgical history, and psychiatric history.

Because ED, low libido, and ejaculatory disorders often have multiple contributing causes, all possible diagnoses must be identified, and a multipronged treatment plan will likely be recommended.

What You Can Do for Yourself

- Talk to your doctor. Don't forget! These issues are common. Your doctor talks to patients about them all the time. Oh . . . and doctors are human, too, struggling with the same issues.
- Be open to their suggestions. Many of the treatments involve psychological treatment. Seeing a therapist is not a sign of weakness. This doesn't mean you are crazy. It's just what we know works!

To improve libido:

- Be open to psychological treatment with psychotherapy, as much of libido is dependent on cognitive arousal.
- Stop marijuana use, and wean off alcohol and narcotic medications with your doctor's guidance.
- Couple's counseling can help rekindle the passion in a relationship.

To improve erectile dysfunction:

- Understand that tactile stimulation becomes more effective at generating an erection than psychologic arousal. Adjust your expectations and activities accordingly.
- Increase overall physical activity.
- Perform weekly sexual activity as it decreases the risk/frequency of ED. This can be accomplished with or without a partner. (Yes, I'm referring to masturbation. I'm not putting any obligations on your partner.)

- In addition to low libido, psychotherapy can help with erectile dysfunction, especially if sensate focus exercises are included.
- Over-the-counter yohimbine may be effective for ED, but the data is limited.
- Some patients will use penis sleeves, which are like hard condoms, or cock rings to stabilize a softer erection to allow for penetration. If you decide to use a cock ring, check with your doctor that it is safe for you to use. Then be sure to use a silicone ring rather than a metal ring, in case you choose a size that is too small. (It is easier to cut off a silicone ring at home and much less embarrassing than having to go to the emergency room to have a metal ring cut off.) You should also use a lot of lubricant, thirty minutes maximum, and trim the hair around the base of the penis shaft to avoid getting the ring caught in the hair. If you want to stimulate your partner as well, consider a cock ring with a vibrator attached.

To treat ejaculatory disorders:

- Behavior and psychological therapy aimed at improving confidence and communication can be very helpful.
- Penile sleeves are like hard condoms that dampen sensation and can be studded to enhance the stimulation of your partner. These are best for patients with premature ejaculation or those who climax earlier than their partner.

What Your Doctor Can Do

To improve libido:

- Recommend psychological treatment with psychotherapy, as much of libido is dependent on cognitive arousal.
- Test your testosterone levels and provide replacement as indicated. Testosterone replacement is indicated ONLY if you are truly deficient (<225ng/dL) on multiple blood laboratory tests drawn between 8 and 10 am; otherwise you can count on testosterone dependency, which causes unpleasant effects on

your mood if you ever have to stop, problems with your blood counts, and then anemia and iron deficiency from a cascade of other treatments. Honestly, young male patients who started testosterone despite having normal levels now have voiced regret for having started testosterone in the first place due to the series of medical complications that they now face.

- Provide access to professional help to stop use of marijuana, alcohol, and narcotic medications.
- If caused by medication, your doctor may be able to decrease the dose or switch to a different medication.

To improve erectile dysfunction:

- If caused by medication, your doctor may be able to decrease the dose or switch to a different medication.
- Diagnose and treat risk factors like smoking, obesity, high blood pressure (hypertension), Type 2 diabetes (diabetes mellitus), and high cholesterol (hyperlipidemia).
- Diagnose and treat sleep apnea.
- Testosterone replacement has only been shown to be beneficial in men who are truly deficient (<225ng/dL) on multiple labs drawn between 8 and 10 am; otherwise, you can count on complications as discussed above.
- Direct treatment options include:
    - PDE5 inhibitors—There are now several on the market: sildenafil (Viagra®) and vardenafil (Levitra®) take sixty minutes to work and last four hours, unless taken daily. Tadalafil (Cialis®) lasts longer at up to thirty-six hours, and avanafil (Stendra®) starts working the quickest, within fifteen minutes of ingestion. They help increase the number and duration of erections. Fortunately for the user, psychological and physical stimulation are required to generate an erection. For fear of sounding like a commercial, please tell your doctor about all of the medications you are taking to avoid severe adverse medication interactions.
    - Vacuum devices—These devices draw blood flow into the penis, and then an occlusive ring, like a cock ring, is used

to keep the blood in the penis longer. While the erection is sufficient for penetration, patients have described the erection as "wet sand in a sock." Of patients, 50 percent continue to use these devices, and 50 percent don't find the resulting erections satisfying.

- Intraurethral alprostadil—This is a cream that is inserted into the urethra and then requires one minute of penile massage to distribute the medication. It tends to be less effective than injections.
- Intracavernosal injections—While the idea makes some squeamish, I do have patients that self-inject alprostadil (Caverject®) into their penises to induce an erection and find this to be their personal ED treatment of choice.
- Penile prosthesis surgery—When the above options fail, some men elect to have prosthetic devices placed. These devices allow for erections to be controlled manually with a pump or button placed inside the scrotum.
- Penile revascularization—This is surgery to divert blood flow, and it is often not recommended for older individuals because the success rate is so poor. I have had some patients successfully complete this surgery, so I would let the surgeon determine if you are a good candidate.

- Separate from low libido, psychotherapy can help with erectile dysfunction, especially if sensate focus exercises are included.
- Currently under investigation are therapies, including stem cell therapy, low-intensity shock therapy (LIST), hyperbaric oxygen therapy, and platelet-rich plasma. Melanocortin receptor agonists and apomorphine have been proven ineffective.

To treat ejaculatory disorders:

- Your doctor may recommend an antidepressant medication in the SSRI category, such as sertraline (Zoloft®), fluoxetine (Prozac®), citalopram (Celexa®), and escitalopram (Lexapro®) as the first-line treatment. While paroxetine (Paxil®) is the most effective, I try to avoid it in the elderly due to other side effects.

- The PDE5 inhibitors may be helpful if concurrent ED (see above).
- Topical anesthetics can help diminish sensation.
- Provide referrals for psychotherapy that can help by both treating the disorder and improving confidence.
- Testosterone is not helpful for ejaculatory disorders.

FDA Warning

There is an FDA warning to protect people from dietary supplements or unapproved prescription drugs sold internationally or illegally that claim to increase penis size, sexual stamina, and performance as 98 percent have been found to be fake, and up to 50 percent have potentially dangerous synthetic chemicals.

Gentleman, I am now going to discuss female sexual dysfunction, but don't just skip to the next chapter; there is more helpful information in just a few paragraphs.

Sexual Dysfunction in Women

Women experience sexual dysfunction as well, and we will focus on the issues that arise with age. With menopause comes a sharp decline in estrogen, and while it is completely normal, most women feel that the loss of estrogen wreaks havoc on their bodies. Menopause occurs when a woman has gone twelve months without a period (menses). The average age of menopause is fifty-one, but the normal range occurs from forty to fifty-eight years old. Perimenopause marks the transition around menopause when hormones are in flux. This time period lasts an average of six years, but the normal range is one to twelve years. Please don't shoot the messenger!

To make this time in our lives more fun, my friends and I decided to have a race to see who would get there first. Who would be the first to go one year without her period? At each gathering, we would announce who was ahead. One friend was ahead at eleven months without her period, until she got it again and had to start back at the starting line.

Checking Bloodwork

When struggling with the symptoms of perimenopause, patients often ask me to check their hormone levels to see if they are getting close to menopause. They want to know how much longer their symptoms are going to last. Unfortunately, there is no test or group of tests that will tell how close a woman is to menopause. Only once menopause has occurred does it become obvious in laboratory testing. At that point, estradiol is virtually nonexistent, and LH and FSH are very high. I will occasionally order these blood tests for women who have had hysterectomies but still have their ovaries and want to know if they are in menopause. Without a uterus, they don't get periods any longer and have no other way of telling if they have officially reached menopause.

Ongoing Consequences of Menopause

With menopause and the subsequent years without estrogen, women experience hot flushes, vaginal atrophy, fatigue, and disruption in sexual function. Hot flushes, also known as hot flashes, occur in 80 percent of women. Fifty percent of women report hot flushes lasting more than seven years. They are often associated with sweating and insomnia. While there are many hypotheses, the cause remains unknown. The reason that I have included hot flushes in this section is that many patients complain that hot flushes disrupt intimacy, occurring every time they hug their intimate partner (and at other times too), making physical closeness unpleasant, frustrating, and sometimes unbearable.

Menopause is a natural part of life that too many women are forced to deal with silently because of cultural norms. One day, I walked into an exam room and immediately felt my face flush and bead up with sweat. As I popped open the buttons on my white coat, I exclaimed, "Thank goodness for hot flushes, usually I'm cold." My fifty-three-year-old female patient laughed and talked about her challenges with menopause. She then thanked me for opening the discussion, for being a "real person," and creating a comfortable environment for a discussion she could never have with her mother or girlfriends. It would be so helpful if moms and daughters discussed menopause, as perimenopausal symptoms and timing of menopause are very heritable and would prepare women for what they are to expect.

My patients have grown to expect my lighthearted, gentle, but direct communication style. However, once, after performing a pelvic exam, I explained to a woman that her vagina was showing signs of what doctors call atrophy. She exclaimed, "Oh, don't say that ugly word!" Well, the good news for her is that the term vaginal atrophy has been renamed genitourinary syndrome of menopause. I, however, find that much harder to say.

With less estrogen, the vaginal mucosa thins and makes less vaginal lubrication. The entrance to the vagina (introitus) shrinks in diameter. The vaginal mucosa becomes pale and smooth, and the cervix and uterus wither. (See Figure 12.1.) Some patients will complain of a sandpaper-like feeling in their vaginal area that is dry, itchy, and burning, with a noticeable change in odor. As an aside, there is also a change in pH that decreases the number of healthy bacteria (lactobacillus) in the vagina, increasing the risk of unhealthy bacteria that cause urinary tract infections. (See Chapter 7.)

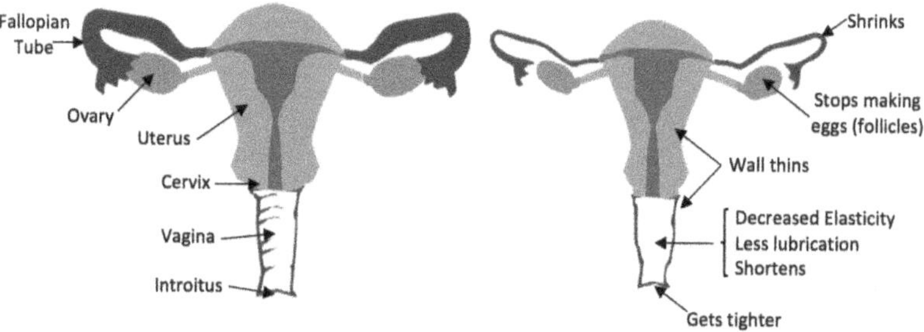

Figure 12.1. A comparison of pre-menopausal female organs and post-menopausal organs.

With age, at least 50 percent of women experience one or more sexual problems. Challenges with sex arise from pain due to decreased lubrication, a narrower entrance to the vagina, prolapsed pelvic organs (see Chapter 9), and decreased libido. Of note, 25 percent of older women are not bothered by their decreased libido, and that is fine, too. Just like men, aging women need more time and stimulation to get aroused, have diminished orgasmic height, and take longer to climax.

What You Can Do for Yourself

To treat and prevent hot flushes:

- Increase hydration—more water again!
- Decrease the ambient temperature by either turning down the heat or turning up the air conditioner and fans.
- Decrease caffeine, alcohol, and spicy food.
- Stop tobacco use (isn't it amazing how many negative health effects tobacco has!).
- Dress in layers and consider dry-weave, moisture-wicking fabrics.
- Replace down comforters with comforters and blankets that are not filled with feathers.
- Slow, deep breathing at the onset of hot flushes diminishes their duration and intensity.
- Fifty minutes of aerobic exercise four days per week, such as walking, running, cycling, and/or swimming, prevents hot flushes.
- Try hypnosis. It has shown benefits.
- Consider acupuncture. It has also demonstrated proven benefits.
- Non-hormone-based supplements such as Estrovera® and Relizen® have data to show their effectiveness. Soy isoflavones, as well as black and red cohosh, have not been found to work in scientific studies.
- An EMBR® wave bracelet is marketed as therapy for hot flashes. I have no experience with it and have not personally heard patient reviews.

What Your Doctor Can Do

- Review medication options such as escitalopram (Lexapro®), venlafaxine (Effexor®), and gabapentin (Neurontin®), which have all been shown to decrease hot flushes.
- Discuss the risks and benefits of hormone replacement therapy for you (see below).

CHAPTER TWELVE

Hormone Replacement Therapy

There is so much information about hormone replacement therapy (HRT) that it can get very confusing for people. To begin, HRT comes in mists, gels, vaginal creams, vaginal tablets, vaginal rings, patches, and pills. I don't really like the mists or gels because then patients have to consider who they are mixing their laundry with and if the mist or gel residue might get on their children or grandchildren. It would be very unhealthy for a boy to be exposed to estrogen products or for girls to be exposed to more estrogen than their bodies are ready for. The other problem is that they are the least well studied. I like vaginal creams, tablets, and rings because the highest concentration of hormones remains (mostly) where you put it, limiting side effects on the rest of the body. Creams are the messiest. Tablets need to be inserted twice weekly. Rings are easy because they stay in for three months at a time. Because the vaginal options only work where you put them, they help with vaginal symptoms, which we will discuss. Unfortunately, they do not help with other symptoms that affect the entire body, like hot flushes or mood swings.

The best things for hot flushes are full-body (systemic) treatments like patches and pills. Patches allow the hormones to get into your system through the skin; therefore, the estrogen isn't processed through the liver, lessening the side effects risk of blood clots. Pills work, too, and for some patients, that is their preferred route of administration, but they are cleared through the liver, so the risk of blood clots is slightly higher. I do not recommend pellets.

Bioidentical hormones are not recommended. I stand in agreement with the North American Menopause Society, American College of Obstetricians and Gynecologists, and the Endocrine Society, which are all against bioidentical hormones. The term itself is misleading. The term *should* refer to a hormone with the same molecular structure as a hormone that your body produces, but in popular culture, as they are sold, it refers to a custom compound of multiple hormones adjusted by a doctor. Secondly, custom compounds lack quality controls regarding purity, and the dosing schedules do not have data to support their use. They are no more or less natural than pharmaceuticals that are also mostly plant-based. Bioidentical hormones like pharmaceuticals also go through a multistep engineering process to be compounded. Lastly, once you get a pellet of hormones inserted, they cannot be removed, so if you develop a negative reaction or a disease that is worsened by these hormones, you have to wait months for them to get out of your system. For example, if you develop a blood clot in your lungs or breast cancer, you can stop a patch or pill, but pellets can't be removed. You may be surprised by my strong stance on this issue and may disagree with me. I respect that. I write from my perspective and experience. In my years of practice, I have seen a lot of irresponsible prescribing of bioidentical hormones and even responsible practices that have put my patients in danger unnecessarily. My goal is to protect you.

Once you decide on the route of administration of your HRT, the next step is to work with your doctor on deciding what hormones should be included. If you choose a vaginal cream or tablet, you will likely only receive an estrogen. If you choose a ring, pill, or patch, then your doctor will need to decide if you also need a progesterone. If you have a uterus, you will want to include progesterone in your HRT to protect the uterine lining and reduce the risk of endometrial cancer. Micronized progesterone is preferred over medroxyprogesterone acetate, but the difference is minimal while the cost is not. If the micronized is too expensive, medroxyprogesterone has been used safely for years.

Some women are prescribed testosterone to help with female sexual function in carefully selected populations and it can help with libido. It does not help with mood, cognition, or hot flushes. If testosterone is prescribed, patients should be maintained within a testosterone range that is normal for women. Too often, I see other doctors provide very high doses of testosterone, placing a woman's hormone levels within male ranges. While this may feel good, I strongly recommend against it as it increases cholesterol, and may increase heart attacks, and strokes, among other things. There is a reason that men, in general, die before women . . . testosterone. In truth, testosterone is rarely needed when all aspects of sexual health are addressed to help with libido.

Here is a brief summary of the risks and benefits of HRT, but please talk to your doctor, who can individualize these risks for you. Estrogens, if started before the age of sixty and within ten years of menopause, increase overall survival for the average woman. They also decrease osteoporosis, hot flushes, skin lesions (but not wrinkles), calcium deposits in the heart, the risk of developing diabetes, and improve blood sugars in the patient who already has diabetes. Estrogens increase vaginal moisture, libido, quality sleep, memory, cognition, and improve mood. For the downside, estrogen alone can cause breast pain like you had before your periods and increase the risk of blood clots, strokes, heartburn, seizures in people with a known seizure disorder, breast cancer, ovarian cancer (a very small risk), and endometrial thickening if you have a uterus and are not taking progesterone. If you add progesterone to the mix, there is an increased risk of breast cancer, especially in women with a body mass index (BMI) <24.4 and those who have breast pain from the HRT, plus worsened mood and migraines. Of note, cancer risks are not lower with bioidentical hormones.

I find that the decision to start HRT is a very personal decision and depends a lot on your personal medical history, the severity of your symptoms and how they impact your life, and your family history. Your doctor can help put the risks and benefits in perspective based on you as an individual.

What You Can Do for Yourself

To treat vaginal atrophy, now called genitourinary syndrome of menopause:

- If your vagina is dry, then use a moisturizer. You moisturize the dry skin on your face, hands, arms, and legs, don't you? Try coconut oil to the vulva (the part of the vagina that you can see on the outside of your body) and a product like Replens® for the vaginal canal.
- Use cleanser rather than soap as it is less drying.
- If you leak urine, use incontinence pads rather than menstrual pads. Consider checking out liquid-absorbing underwear like Speax® by Thinx.
- Stop shaving your pubic hair (if you do) as it helps keep the vagina moist. Trim the hair instead if you prefer a manicured appearance.
- Limit intimate wipes as they, too, are very drying.
- Exercise (really???). There are studies to suggest that intercourse with a penis, a dildo, or a vibrator delays atrophy, stimulates blood flow, gland production of lubrication, and keeps the vaginal canal open. I'm often asked if the studies were conducted by men . . . but I do agree with their conclusions. I've seen patients struggle to get function back after a

hiatus from sexual intercourse, which, of course, is possible but takes more effort.

What Your Doctor Can Do

To treat vaginal atrophy, now called genitourinary syndrome of menopause:

- Prescribe estrogen vaginal cream, estradiol vaginal tablets, or a vaginal estrogen ring (which, coincidentally, can also help with overactive bladder—see Chapter 8).

What You Can Do for Yourself

Tips to assist with sexual function:

- Maintain your vaginal health as above between sexual activity.
- Because the clitoris becomes less sensitive with time, it may need more stimulation to become engorged and for women to climax. Consider adding sex toys to your repertoire. Many partners feel like vibrators and dildos are competition or a sign that they are failing in their performance. Nonsense. Toys can be a part of playful exploration between you and your partner and should not be perceived as a threat. They are completely different and allow for a different sensation, not replacing the warmth or intimacy of another individual.
- Use lubricants. I recommend Astroglide gel® for my patients, and it is also one of the least irritating. Water-based lubricants are preferred. Silicone-based lubricants can damage other silicone products such as toys and medical devices like dilators and HRT rings. Oil-based lubricants are associated with higher rates of infection and torn condoms.
- Because the opening of the vagina shrinks, consider stretching the vaginal canal prior to penetration. This can be done with your or your partner's fingers. Start by inserting one lubed finger into the vagina, then once the vagina has had a chance to stretch, remove the finger and try inserting two. If you prefer, you can use a lubricated dildo prior to intercourse instead.

Make it a new form of foreplay. Then, at the start of intercourse, after initial penetration, wait and allow the vagina to stretch before engaging in any movement or thrusting activity.

- If the vagina still needs more stretching or is experiencing pain, see your doctor, and they may recommend graduated dilators to stretch the vagina and/or to ease vaginal spasms. Dilators are silicone tube-shaped devices of increasing size that can be inserted into the vagina twice a week to help with vaginal pain and muscle spasms.
- Constipation can interfere with sexual comfort, so be sure to treat your bowels. (See Chapter 11.)
- If your uterus has dropped over time from numerous or large childbirths, deep vaginal penetration will become more difficult and painful. Look into Ohnuts. They are soft rings that can be placed on a penis or dildo to serve as a bumper, limiting the distance of penetrance while transmitting sensation down the remainder of the unpenetrated penis.
- If there is enough room in the vagina, other devices that increase stimulation for both partners are called couples vibrators, such as the We-Vibe Sync.

What Your Doctor Can Do

Tips to assist with sexual function:

- If the vaginal opening remains too tight despite the measures above, a doctor can clip open the introitus. It sounds terrible . . . I've heard that it is quick and not too uncomfortable.
- Botox® can also relax the muscles if muscle spasms are worsening pain with intercourse.
- Your doctor may discuss medications depending on the reason for sexual dysfunction, including SSRIs such as fluoxetine (Prozac®), Escitalopram (Lexapro®), citalopram (Celexa®), sertraline (Zoloft®), gabapentin (Neurontin®), or nortriptyline (Pamelor®).

- Pelvic physical therapy is also beneficial for many people and can be more helpful than Kegel exercises alone. Your doctor may give you a referral.
- A doctor may also have to address any prolapsed organs (see Chapter 9).

What You Can Do for Yourself

Looking for assistance with libido?

- Be open to psychological treatment with psychotherapy, as much of libido is dependent on cognitive arousal.
- Stop marijuana use and wean off alcohol and narcotic medications with your doctor's guidance.
- Couple's counseling can help rekindle the passion in a relationship.

What Your Doctor Can Do

Looking for assistance with libido?

- Discuss estrogen patches or pills with your doctor, as they can help (remember, if you have a uterus, you must take progesterone as well).
- Testosterone can help, especially if serum levels are less than eight, but heed the warnings about not taking too much (see above).
- PDE5 inhibitors such as sildenafil (Viagra®), vardenafil (Levitra®), tadalafil (Cialis®), and avanafil (Stendra®) enlarge the clitoris but don't necessarily help libido. They can be beneficial in women with nerve damage to the vaginal area (i.e., from multiple sclerosis or from spinal cord injuries).
- Antidepressants bupropion (Wellbutrin®) or buspirone (Buspar®) have shown benefits in improving libido.
- There is a new option, though not necessarily highly recommended, called bremelanotide (Vyleesi®). It is an injection that increases feelings of desire and lowers distress around

having sex but has only a modest effect on increasing the number of sexually satisfying encounters.

Sex Should Be Fun

Don't forget that sex is fun. Choose a safe person and enjoy whatever you are able to do. Make sure both partners feel comfortable and are enjoying the experience. Sexually transmitted diseases are not different as you age, so I didn't spend much time talking about them. But if you have a new sexual partner, you can both get tested prior to sexual activity. You can also use condoms. I mentioned testing first because condoms become harder to wear as men age. They make it more challenging to maintain an erection, and hand arthritis makes them harder to put on. Also, if you talk to your doctor about testing, then your doctor can talk to you about vaccinations and preventative medications, depending on your sexual practices. If you think you have a sexually transmitted infection, don't hesitate to talk to your doctor. You won't be the first or the last . . . that week. We are here to help you, want to keep you healthy, and want you to be able to feel fulfilled in this aspect of your life. Sex should be a positive experience in your life.

Sex and Intimacy Doesn't Need to Stop

Too often, I see patients who reflect and lament over the loss of intimacy because their partner can no longer perform sexually. They want intimacy more than having a sexual experience like they were twenty years old again. Their partner is withdrawn romantically as they struggle. Either they are afraid to get help or are so ashamed that they give up on intimacy altogether.

If you or your partner cannot engage in sexual activity, don't lose that very significant part of your life too. Work together on intimacy and romance. Be creative, and continue to pleasure the able person in new ways or allow them to masturbate and fulfill that need for themselves. Sex is a healthy part of life and provides a wonderful sense of vitality. Everyone benefits physically, mentally, and spiritually from closeness and the chemical releases that occur with all levels of intimacy. Don't give that up if it hasn't been taken from you. Even a six-second hug releases the feel-good hormone oxytocin!

Before you begin a conversation with your doctor, remember that doctors are human too. We carry insecurities about our bodies and what they can and can't do. I sure hope you can find a doctor with whom, in the privacy and confidentiality of an office visit, you can talk about anything and everything without embarrassment or shame . . . including sexual dysfunction. Your entire body and well-being deserve great medical care so that you can live a deeply meaningful life.

CHAPTER THIRTEEN

INSOMNIA: ONE SHEEP, TWO SHEEP, THREE SHEEP . . .

Insomnia Is Common

Darn it! I will not sleep until I find a cure for insomnia! Why? Because I'm in deep trouble. Every week that I am on call, I'm afraid that my spouse is going to make me sleep in the doghouse. With each ring of my phone from a patient in need, I wake up, leave the bedroom, address the concern, return to the bed, curl up in the blankets, and fall immediately back to sleep. One of the benefits of my medicine residency training was learning how to turn sleep on and off like a light switch. My spouse did not complete a residency and has not had to learn that skill. Now, jolted from a deep sleep by the phone, she lays in bed for hours staring at the ceiling, trying to calm her nerves and settle her heart rate, desperately hoping for an ounce of sleep before the morning alarm rings or the dogs and cat start begging for breakfast.

At least half of my patients over the age of fifty have come to me with complaints of insomnia. Sleep is so important as this is the time that we consolidate memories, process information from the day, and our brains go into a self-cleaning mode, as cerebral spinal fluid flushes toxins from the brain. I find that younger patients have trouble falling asleep while older patients have more trouble staying asleep. Older patients who struggle with sleep maintenance, as doctors call it, fall asleep fine only to wake up at 2 am unable to return to slumber. (Yes, my spouse is over fifty . . . but if I say by how much, I might be headed to divorce court.) In the worst cases of insomnia, patients get their sleep cycle reversed, sleeping during the day while being awake all night.

The Regulation of Sleep

In the brain, the suprachiasmatic nucleus (SCN) within the hypothalamus controls our twenty-four-hour daily internal clock, called our circadian rhythm. This rhythm affects when we wake up and go to sleep, when we eat, and when hormones are released in our bodies. Aging affects the function of the SCN, disrupting the circadian rhythm. All hormone production decreases with age, but it is the decrease in melatonin and cortisol production that further disrupts sleep quality.

The SCN also needs adequate daylight exposure to function properly, which many seniors do not get. As the body is exposed to daylight, it makes melatonin, causing the amount of melatonin in our bodies to rise throughout the day. When melatonin reaches a certain elevated level, it signals to the body that it is time to go to sleep. Sleep causes the melatonin levels to drop so that the cycle can begin the next day again. Long naps in the middle of the day cause melatonin levels to drop prematurely, altering the quality of night sleep, because melatonin is then not able to rise to high enough levels again prior to bedtime.

It is natural for patients to want to go to bed earlier and rise earlier as they age. When they do sleep, they spend more time in the earlier and lighter stages of sleep (Stage 1 and 2) and less time in the deeper stages (Stage 3 and 4), making it more likely that they will be awoken in the night or else feel like they had a restless night of sleep. Daytime napping is a great idea to make up for lost sleep as older individuals need the same amount of sleep as middle-aged adults, which is seven to eight hours per night. However, extended daytime napping can interfere with the quality of night sleep, as previously discussed.

With age, patients tend to accumulate diseases and medications that can disrupt sleep. Osteoarthritis alone makes it difficult for patients to get comfortable, and it causes pain and stiffness that disrupt sleep. Enlarging prostates and weak pelvic floor muscles lead to frequent nighttime urination. Limited vision and poor mobility make trips to the bathroom more disruptive to sleep. Unlike when you were thirty years old, each trip requires you to be more awake. You need to turn on lights so that you can see to prevent falls. You will walk slower and spend more time out of bed to accomplish your task, taking you further from your dreamy state. Sadness from isolation and loss may make it harder to fall back to sleep as the mind starts to wander. Consequences of medications may cause daytime drowsiness or disrupt sleep at night. Other diseases, like obstructive sleep apnea, restless leg syndrome, and REM sleep behavior disorder, where people act out their dreams, all increase episodes of wakefulness as one is trying to get a restful night's sleep.

Without Restful Sleep

Without a good night's sleep, people feel daytime fatigue, malaise, increased forgetfulness, have poor attention, diminished concentration, irritability, low energy, make mistakes, and have ongoing worry about sleep. Your doctor may order a sleep study (polysomnography) to rule out treatable sleep disorders, such as obstructive sleep apnea or periodic limb movement of sleep. Fortunately, sleep studies can be done at home rather than in a lab, which most patients find more appealing.

What You Can Do for Yourself

- Open your blinds every day and close them at night. Expose yourself to daylight throughout the day, every day.
- Exercise regularly. It will both help you fall asleep faster and help you sleep longer and deeper.
- No blue screens two hours before bed. Blue screens are found in most flat screens, like newer flat-screen televisions, computers, tablets, and phones.
- Remove televisions and computers from the bedroom. If you have a cellphone in the bedroom, only use it for emergencies.
- Avoid anything that disrupts sleep: alcohol, tobacco, caffeine, large meals late in the day, and/or excessively long naps in the day or early evening. Caution: caffeine is hidden in many foods, beverages, and certain medications, so read labels and avoid these products.
- Go to sleep at the same time and wake up at the same time every day.

- Make your sleep environment comfortable.
- Use your bed only for sleep and sex.
- Anyone who knows me knows how hard it is for me to say this, but you must keep the pets off the bed. While they may help you fall asleep, they can be terribly disruptive to sleep maintenance.
- Do not have a clock that is directly visible from where you lie in bed, as clock-watching increases anxiety.
- Develop a bedtime ritual. For example, I brush and floss my teeth, wash and lotion my face, take my medication, put on my pajamas, stretch for twenty minutes, make one last attempt at emptying my bladder, and take my teddy bear with me to bed (did I just admit that to the world?).
    - Other ideas: write about your day, read, think of three things that you are grateful for, acknowledge your wins for the day, play a game (no video/screen), sleep meditation, calming yoga, saying thanks, repetitive acts like knitting, take a bath.
- Make sure you have enough pillows to prop yourself up to ease pain.
- Consider mindful practices like meditation, mantra repetition, and self-massage to help yourself relax if you find yourself awake.
- Some people like the smell of lavender to promote sleep.
- Before trying prescription medications, try over-the-counter products like melatonin, valerian, and/or teas like Sleepy Time® tea by Celestial Seasonings or Bedtime Tea® by Yogi, or magnesium. Some of my patients really like Calmme® by Mason. Diphenhydramine is NOT recommended in the aging adult as it has side effects that cause brain fogginess that can lead to injury and may make it difficult for men to urinate.
- I do live in Colorado, where marijuana is readily available, and some of my patients use it for sleep. While I have recommended topical CBD for arthritic joints, I discourage my older patients from using marijuana products that are ingested or inhaled as I've seen an increased rate of falls with injury,

disorientation, and confusion among patients using marijuana, especially before bed.

- Avoid combining sleep medications with alcohol, opioid pain medication, or other sedatives, which will magnify the side effects and risks.
- Be sure to discuss the risks of all sleep medications, prescription or otherwise, with your doctor.

What Your Doctor Can Do

- Refer you for cognitive behavioral therapy (CBT). CBT is the preferred first line of treatment for chronic insomnia because it works better than medications. Unfortunately, this may not be an option for everyone due to availability of qualified therapists, resources to pay for therapy, or cognitive ability to participate meaningfully.
- Test you for underlying conditions that may be affecting your sleep, including ordering an at-home sleep study
- Treat underlying conditions that may be affecting your sleep
- For patients who have trouble falling asleep, where it takes more than thirty minutes to fall asleep, but once asleep they generally stay asleep, your doctor may consider medications like zolpidem (Ambien®), eszopiclone (Lunesta®), zaleplon (Sonata®), ramelteon (Rozerem®), lemborexant (Dayvigo®), suvorexant (Belsomra®), and trazodone
- For patients who have trouble staying asleep, your doctor may discuss low-dose doxepin (Silenor®), lemborexant (Dayvigo®), suvorexant (Belsomra®), trazodone, or gabapentin (Neurontin®) with you
- Some of the medications work for both falling asleep and staying asleep. If one medication treats two problems, I often try to choose those so as to limit pill burden. For example, if a patient needs help with sleep and an appetite stimulant, my first choice is mirtazapine (Remeron®). At higher doses, mirtazapine brightens one's mood, too.
- For the same reason that I don't like marijuana for sleep in the elderly, I prefer not to use benzodiazepines like alprazolam

(Xanax®), diazepam (Valium®), or lorazepam (Ativan®). All medications with generic names that end in "-pam" increase the risk of falls, confusion, excessive sedation, delirium, and balance problems. These are side effects that can be catastrophic in the elderly. Older adults are at increased risk of side effects as the medications stay in the body longer and at higher medication levels (see Chapter 17).

- Again . . . because it is really important! Avoid combining sleep medications with alcohol, opioid pain medication, or other sedatives that will magnify the side effects and risks. If you are trying new sleep medication, check your alertness, memory, and coordination the next day, before you get behind the wheel of a car. Your doctor can review all of the risks and benefits of these medications with you.

Gifts of Insomnia

Please don't throw rotten tomatoes. I am a good sleeper, but I do know what it feels like to be tired to the core. In my three years of residency, I lost the equivalent of six months of sleep given all of the thirty-plus-hour shifts and extra shifts to pay my monthly student loan payments. After a long shift with no sleep, my body ached, my head hurt, my body craved carbohydrates, and I felt like I was being propelled forward not by my own free will but by brief surges of adrenaline.

Now, I am a wife, daughter, sister, aunt, mother of fuzzy four-legged children, a physician, a friend, a neighbor, an academic, a writer, a public speaker, a struggling athlete, a baker of mostly pies, a gardener, a reader, a continuous student of medicine, a community participant, and a patient. I have everything I ever wanted in my life except enough time to be creative. When I find myself awake in bed, I never fret. I am grateful for that time to just be still and to think, with no distractions, and to just be with myself. It is such a peaceful time. I went about twenty years of my life, where the only moment of true peace I got was the twenty minutes I had snuck away from the hospital to lie on an MRI table. Now I relish the time that I am just barely rested enough to be actually awake at night, all by myself, yet comforted by the low incongruous rumbles of dogs snoring on their beds on the floor and the soft breathing of my spouse.

How can you turn your awake moments into treasures? Or at least not moments of turmoil that lead to frustration and more insomnia? Which of these tips are most helpful for reducing the causes of your insomnia?

Now you might be asking yourself, "If Dr. Guerrasio is such a good doctor, why does her spouse struggle to fall back asleep after being awoken?" Not every day goes as planned. Some days, she doesn't get any exercise after sitting all day for work. She likes to read off of her blue-screen phone until the exact moment in bed before she turns out the lights. She drinks an occasional Colorado craft stout beer or glass of wine with dinner. And when I'm gone, she lets the BIG lab-shepherd mix sleep on my side of the bed. When it comes down to it, we all have our priorities. Sometimes, there are right and wrong answers, and sometimes there are competing values. Life is a balancing act, and that balancing act becomes more complex with age. Somedays, it is more important to her to catch up on the news in bed, relax with a beverage, and snuggle with her protective dog. Other days, sleep is her priority. How wonderful to have the choice and ability to adjust our behaviors to vary the outcomes!

CHAPTER FOURTEEN
DIZZINESS: ROUND AND ROUND AND UP THEN DOWN

Amusement Rides

When I was growing up, I had what I refer to as my twin cousin. My cousin Janice and I were the same age, shared some similar physical characteristics, grew up in the same area of New York, had similar friends, went to the same public schools, and were in the same grade. When we were in high school, if Janice and I went to an amusement park, we would run in opposite directions. Janice loved the roller coasters—the really tall roller coasters with upside-down loops. The steepest drops were her favorite. I loved the rides that spun you in circles until you could no longer walk in a straight line. After consecutive rides, we would leave the parks both dizzy, but our experiences of dizziness were different. Mostly because we had been shaken in different directions. You might say my dizziness was more like vertigo and hers more like lightheadedness.

Likewise, patients experience what they call dizziness in many different ways. For some people, dizziness means feeling lightheaded or faint, as if you might pass out. For others, dizziness is the sensation that your environment is moving or spinning around you. Doctors refer to this as vertigo. Both are very common among aging individuals (and they don't even have to ride roller coasters!), and we will explore both separately.

CHAPTER FOURTEEN

Lightheadedness

I spent many years working at a hospital that was adjacent to a golf course. Every summer, I would admit multiple patients to the geriatric ward for lightheadedness (pre-syncope) and/or passing out (syncope). The story often went like this: Sam, an eighty-two-year-old man, decided to go golfing one August morning. Because he didn't want to urinate during the outing, Sam would either eat a small breakfast and skip a drink or skip breakfast altogether. Then, by hole four, the day would turn out to be warmer than he expected and the sun brighter than forecasted. Before long, Sam would begin to feel beads of sweat on his forehead followed by a feeling of lightheadedness, then by narrowing of his vision. If he got to his water bottle in time, he might avoid a trip to the emergency room for dehydration and urgent need for intravenous (IV) fluids. Many people who tempted fate during the summer months, under the blazing sun and in the dry climate, did not fare well, and they would be escorted via sirens and flashing lights to the hospital to be evaluated for dizziness and/or loss of consciousness.

This type of dizziness is most often caused by dehydration but can also be caused by a sudden drop in blood pressure, low blood sugar, an irregular heartbeat (arrhythmia), electrolyte abnormalities, medications, and anxiety. Approximately one-third of older adults experience lightheadedness, and there are many reasons that elderly people are predisposed to lightheadedness. First, elderly people are chronically dehydrated at baseline and need much more water to stay hydrated. As people get older, their thirst sensation or thirst craving greatly diminishes, so they can't tell when they are dehydrated, and they just aren't aware to drink enough fluids. Also, the kidneys are unable to concentrate urine as well, so that older people lose a lot of extra water, urinating out a very dilute urine. It doesn't stop there. Further compounding the problem, access to water also decreases as limited mobility makes getting a drink more difficult or even impossible.

Normally, when one stands up, their heart rate increases, and their blood vessels clamp down to push blood towards the brain, but with age, this response is less effective. The heart rate cannot augment to the same degree as the maximum heart rate is lower with each year. When the heart rate does increase, it changes more slowly. Why, you ask? This is because the adrenal glands make fewer hormones, like adrenaline and norepinephrine, and the heart has fewer receptors to receive the hormones circulating in the blood. Access to these hormones is needed to maximize your heart rate and quickly. Now the blood vessels also have a delayed response and are less effective at squeezing blood back to the brain because, over time, the vessels get calcified and are less pliable. They just don't squeeze as well. All of these limitations contribute to the increased risk of lightheadedness.

As for the other causes of lightheadedness, bodily systems that regulate blood sugar become more fragile with age, so blood sugars become more labile, trending up and down erratically and more quickly. Low blood sugars and dropping blood sugars can cause lightheadedness. Blood sugars are also regulated by a hormonal system that experiences a decline in hormone production. With less activity at the receptor sites, communication from chemical messengers to correct blood sugars is impaired.

Scarring in the heart's conduction system from age can cause low heart rates (heart block and sick sinus syndrome). The rhythm of your heart is electrical and is conducted along pathways that look a lot like a county map. Your heart essentially has a highway of wires that conduct the electricity from top to bottom then to the sides. If the highway of wires gets damaged, such as by scar tissue over the years, the heart must rely on a backup system. There are several backup systems in place that include different on-ramps where the electrical signal can start. If the highway is closed altogether, the electricity must take the side streets, communicating cell by cell, but that process is much slower and would eventually require a pacemaker to replace the highway.

Dehydration and a diminished intake of food can lead to electrolyte abnormalities, a low-sodium concentration in particular. This does not necessarily mean that adding salt to your food would make your dizziness better, as the problem is not the total amount of sodium in your body but rather the ratio between sodium and water. You will need your doctor's input to help you determine if you need more or less water and/or salt added to your diet. This is much more complicated than it sounds.

Medications are more likely to cause unexpected changes in blood sugar, blood pressure, and electrolytes abnormalities in the elderly because people become more sensitive to medication side effects as they age (see Chapter 17). Visual and hearing impairments exacerbate lightheadedness as they contribute to disorientation (see Chapter 18). This is not meant to be an exhaustive list but just to help you better understand how the body changes with the aging process and that many factors contribute to lightheadedness.

What You Can Do for Yourself

- Talk to your doctor about your symptoms so that he or she can review the cause of your lightheadedness and the best treatment strategy.
- Most lightheadedness can be prevented by drinking plenty of fluids every day and eating balanced healthy meals throughout the day.
- Avoid very hot weather.
- Stand up slowly. If you are lying down, first sit on the edge of the bed for a few seconds and then stand for a few seconds before you start walking.
- If you are experiencing lightheadedness, first sit down on the floor so that in case you pass out, you won't fall and hurt yourself.
- If you are a diabetic, have someone check your blood sugar to see if it is too low.
- See your doctor regularly to have an exam and to have your medications adjusted and bloodwork checked.

What Your Doctor Can Do

- Help you determine the cause of your lightheadedness. They may draw your labs to check your blood work, place a heart monitor on you, or perform an EKG to evaluate your heart rhythm. They may recommend drinking more water, may give you IV fluids, recommend electrolytes, or to eat or drink something sugary when you feel lightheaded.
- Depending on the cause, some people need water pills, like furosemide (Lasix®).
- Some need a low-salt diet, while others need to add salt to their diet.
- Some need the head of their bed raised, and others need compression stockings.

- Yet some might need psychotherapy or anxiety medicine.
- Because the treatments are so varied for the different causes of lightheadedness, it is most important that you speak to your doctor.

Vertigo

In my clinical practice, I often have patients complain of dizziness, sometimes associated with severe nausea. Jill is a classic case. She is a seventy-five-year-old woman who rolls over in bed and all of a sudden the room starts to spin. She becomes very nauseated and is afraid she will vomit. She doesn't know why because she felt fine when she went to bed and reports sleeping fairly well. When she tries to sit up in bed, the spinning or vertigo gets worse. Anytime she moves her head, the symptoms get worse! And it is a horribly incapacitating feeling.

Let's take a look at the ear (see Figure 14.1). The ear has three parts: the outer ear, which amplifies sound; the middle ear, which turns sound waves into vibrations; and the inner ear, which both changes these vibrations into electrical signals and interprets your position in space. Specifically, the semicircular canals consist of three tiny tubes lined with tiny hairs that are filled with fluid. Tiny calcium carbonate crystals called otoconia move in the utricle and saccule, which are also lined with tiny hairs. When the head is moved, the fluid inside the canals, utricle, and saccule moves, causing the otoconia to roll around, bending the hairs. As the hairs bend, they are signaling to the brain that the body has moved, which direction, how fast, and where the body is in space.

With age, the crystals become roughened, fractured, and hollow through a process of demineralization. While there is some controversy over exactly how this change increases vertigo with aging, maneuvers to reposition the crystals are an effective way to improve symptoms. Some speculate that these abnormal crystals are more likely to get stuck in one place and interfere with the drainage of fluid from the utricle or the semicircular canals. If this happens, a person will perceive the world around them spinning, then get nauseated, possibly vomit, feel unsteady on their feet, and have difficulty walking. Unfortunately, recurrent episodes are common. With certain types of vertigo, you can have blurred vision, difficulty speaking, and hearing loss. All of these symptoms require urgent

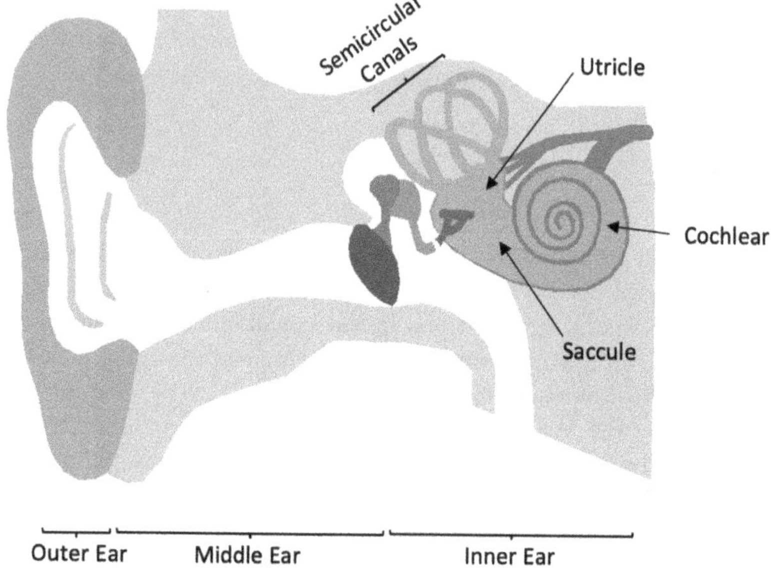

Figure 14.1. Anatomy of the inner ear.

evaluation to ensure that you are not having a stroke. These episodes can last seconds or even days.

If you present to your doctor with vertigo, they will ask about the time course, aggravating and provoking factors, associated symptoms, and review your prior medical history. Unfortunately, the diagnostic examination for vertigo is designed to elicit symptoms. The specific symptom that your doctor is looking for is called nystagmus. Nystagmus is a very unique, repetitive, involuntary eye movement, where the eye almost shakes back and forth like an exaggerated vibration or pendulum at high speed. The doctor may also check your balance, how you walk, and test your hearing with tuning forks or, more formally, with audiometry. Expect the doctor to move you around quite a bit. They will perform a Dix-Hallpike maneuver, having you sit, look to one side, and lie down while they watch your eyes. You will be asked to repeat this while looking in the opposite direction. A head impulse test may also be conducted where you are asked to look forward and the doctor turns your head left and right. Most patients don't need more sophisticated tests like an MRI, electronystagmography, video nystagmography, vestibular evoked myogenic potential, and brainstem auditory evoked potentials. These tests are not standardized, nor are they widely available for clinical use. That is for your doctor to decide.

While there are many causes of vertigo, those most related to age are benign paroxysmal positional vertigo (BPPV) and Meniere's disease. If your doctor determines that the cause is from BPPV, the treatment is the Epley maneuver. First, the doctor will perform the Dix-Hallpike maneuver mentioned above to determine which ear is affected. If it is your right ear that is affected, the doctor will have you lie on your back with your head rotated forty-five degrees to the right. You will be asked to lie there for thirty to forty seconds, then you will rotate your head forty-five degrees to the left for thirty to forty seconds. Next, you will roll onto your left shoulder, keeping your head turned forty-five degrees to the left for thirty to forty seconds. At this point, you will be looking toward the ground. Finally, you will sit up with your legs dangling off the left side of the bed, looking forward for thirty to forty seconds. The maneuver may need to be repeated.

For chronic management of vertigo, to reduce the number and severity of attacks, I have had success sending patients to a special kind of physical therapy called vestibular rehabilitation. A very small number of people with intractable symptoms are treated with surgery or argon lasers.

Meniere's disease is distinct from BPPV as patients also develop ringing in one or both ears (tinnitus) that may occur with or separate from the vertigo, hearing loss, and a sensation of ear fullness. Dietary recommendations include reducing intake of the following: salt, caffeine, alcohol, nicotine, stress, and/or monosodium glutamate (MSG). There is data to suggest control of environmental and food allergies also helps. During an attack, the current recommendations are to use meclizine with or without a benzodiazepine such as clonazepam at the lowest possible dose for the vertigo. Promethazine or ondansetron can be used for the nausea.

For chronic management, to reduce the number and severity of attacks, I also recommend vestibular rehabilitation between attacks for Meniere's disease as for BPPV. Mild water pills (diuretics) like hydrochlorothiazide and triamterene can also help prevent attacks. Unfortunately, there is no high-quality data on the efficacy of these medications, although they are used widely. If symptoms just don't stop, there are steroid and surgical options available.

Currently, there is no convincing data to support the use of medications that suppress the immune system, like methotrexate or etanercept, or positive pressure pulse generators to help with vertigo. There are also no convincing studies that vitamins or herbal remedies affect vertigo despite promotions of ginkgo biloba (which can increase risks of bleeding), ginger tea, and almonds for vertigo in general.

What You Can Do

- Ask your doctor to determine what type of vertigo you have, and this may include a hearing test.
- If you have BPPV, learn how to do the Epley maneuver. One of my favorite videos demonstrating the maneuver was produced by Fauquier ENT and is available on YouTube at: https://www.youtube.com/watch?v=9SLm76jQg3g&t=26s; you can also type Epley Maneuver to Treat BPPV Vertigo into the YouTube search field.
- You may need to repeat this maneuver on yourself from time to time. Once the diagnosis is established, you will find it easier to do this at home than to drive to the doctor to have it done. Being in the car while you are feeling nauseated is most unpleasant.
- If you have Meniere's disease, reduce salt and stress and eliminate caffeine, alcohol, nicotine, and MSG from your life!
- Ask your doctor about vestibular rehabilitation. Not all physical therapists have the specialized equipment to perform this type of therapy. You will need to be referred to a specific rehabilitation facility.
- If you have had an attack before, keep vertigo and anti-nausea medications on hand for subsequent attacks.

What Your Doctor Can Do

- Determine the type of vertigo you have and make sure that you are not having a stroke! Vertigo from strokes is very rare but important not to miss.
- Order a hearing test (audiometry).
- Perform the Dix-Hallpike and Epley maneuvers on you.

- Prescribe medication like meclizine with or without a benzodiazepine such as clonazepam at the lowest possible dose for the vertigo and promethazine or ondansetron for the nausea.
- If you have BPPV and symptoms persist, surgery and laser procedures may be recommended, but this is rare.
- For Meniere's disease, your doctor may also prescribe hydrochlorothiazide and triamterene to prevent recurrent attacks.

Doesn't it seem like I always manage to squeeze some form of exercise into every chapter? This time instead of recommending exercise in general, I have you rolling around on a table or bed to move crystals. Such effort sounds like minimal exercise to some, but for people with arthritis or who don't move easily, it can be a feat.

Medicine Is Full of Magic

Honestly, this is one of the more fulfilling moments that I have had as a doctor. Greater than 80 percent of my patients who come to the office with lightheadedness or vertigo leave feeling dramatically better when they leave. It's like magic! Either fluid fixes the dehydration or the Epley maneuver works like magic, and they leave feeling stable on their feet once again. I know that magicians aren't supposed to give away their secrets. They should make everything seem like an illusion behind the mysterious curtain, under the spellbinding chant, or inside the mysterious box. I am willing to be a terrible magician by revealing my secrets, if it makes just one person feel better or if it makes just one person's life easier. Fluids or an Epley maneuver may not seem very magical to the skeptic, but then, how magical is a mirror really? As a patient, I prefer to believe in the mirror and the devotion of the magician.

CHAPTER FIFTEEN
LOWER LEG SWELLING: STILL A ROSE TO ME

Leg Swelling Changes Everything

While I personally don't carry this sentiment, I grew up in a family that was against tattoos. No one had them. Not my parents, grandparents, nor my immediate aunts and uncles. The first time I remember meeting my great-aunt Gertrude, I was probably five years old. She had come to a summer backyard barbeque at our house for a family gathering and was wearing a frilly yellow summer dress. She gave me a big, soft, full hug and commented on my swinging pigtails. She hobbled across the grass with her eighty-five-year-old legs to a nearby lawn chair and sat down. And there it was, the first tattoo I had ever seen up close. It was just above the right knee of her thick legs, with swollen calves and ankles.

"Aunt Gert!" I shouted in all of my childhood wonder and excitement, "You have a tattoo of a duck!"

While my mother was mortified, Aunt Gertrude gently pulled at her sagging leg to stretch out her skin and the tattoo of what I thought was a duck, instead revealing what was a beautiful old tattoo of a rose.

"Well, it used to be a rose," she laughed, "but the color is gone, and I suppose it does now look more like a duck. Let me tell you about the dresses I used to wear when I was a flapper and had skinny young legs like yours!"

From then on, she became my rose as I learned more about what it meant to her to have been a flapper in the 1920s and how she ended up with her special tattoo.

Her legs had stretched and shrunk so many times from what is called edema that the skin had gotten looser over time. That day her thighs were loose, and the calves were tight, but I would eventually see the thighs full of water and tight other days, allowing me to admire her brave rose tattoo! The heavy swelling in her legs affected her ability to walk, move around, sit, and rest comfortably. The medications that helped reduce the swelling also kept her tied close to a bathroom. Of course, I realized none of this at the time, nor did I even question it. They were just Aunt Gertrude's legs.

Definition of Edema

Our blood vessels circulate blood throughout our bodies, but they are not as waterproof as you might imagine. Blood vessels are leaky. The walls of your blood vessels are made up of cells lined end to end, and fluid under pressure can push its way out between these cells. This escaped fluid ends up in the space between the tissues outside of the blood vessels. This causes swelling that doctors call edema. Unequal pressure between the fluid in the blood vessel and the tissues outside of the blood vessels is one way to develop swelling. You can also develop swelling if you are malnourished and there isn't enough protein inside of the blood vessels to help draw the fluid in (via an osmotic gradient), and lastly, if you have an injury, your body will intentionally send inflammatory cells to that area to treat the injury resulting in swelling (see Figure 15.1).

Understanding Why Edema Happens

Let's look at unequal pressure first. All day long, this edema, the fluid outside of the blood vessels, is pulled down towards your legs by gravity. When you go to bed and raise your legs, the fluid is able to move back into the bloodstream and circulate to the kidneys. Once at the kidneys, you are able to urinate out any excess fluid. This explains why people make more urine at night. In addition to elevating the legs, exercise, even as simple as walking, moves muscles that help push the edema back into the blood vessels. Thus, any excess fluid can be circulated to the kidneys and urinated out of the

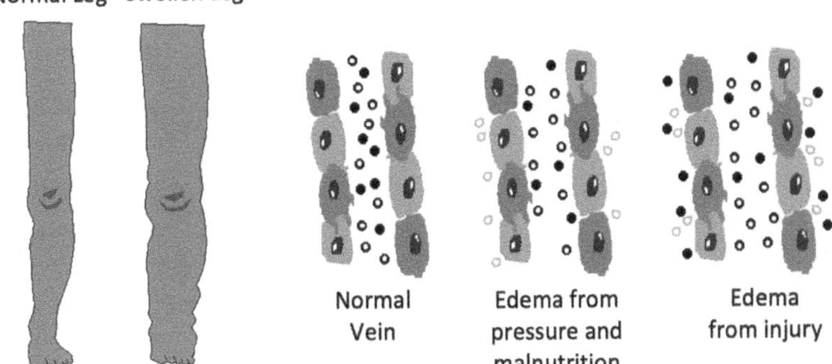

Figure 15.1. Blood vessels and the different ways they can leak and cause swelling.

body. If you are walking and exercising less, you are more likely to develop edema. Think about what happens to your feet and ankles if you sit on an airplane for hours. They swell, and your shoes feel tight.

Now, if your heart isn't pumping very strongly (heart failure or an irregular heartbeat/arrhythmia), then the fluid can't get to the kidney to be urinated out of the body. And it ends up pooling in the legs. This creates undue pressure in the blood vessels, causing fluid to leak out into the surrounding tissues. If the kidneys are failing and aren't able to urinate out enough fluid, that can also cause edema because blood pools in the legs. Once again, as the pressure builds up in the blood vessels, fluid leaks out into the surrounding tissue. In medical school, I learned over and over again that water follows salt, so the more salt you eat, the more excess fluid will build up in your blood vessels, creating that same pressure that causes leakage. If you develop a blood clot in one leg, pressure will build up behind that "dam," just like a clogged waterway or pipe, and edema will occur in the one leg below the clot. Since the blocked vein will not allow blood to return as efficiently to the heart, blood will pool, and edema will develop.

If you are malnourished from a poor diet, have a failing liver that can no longer make enough protein, or have faltering kidneys that urinate out too much protein, you will also develop edema. This edema tends to affect the entire body, worse in areas of the body most affected by gravity, like the legs when sitting and standing and the buttock when reclining. In this case, the leakage occurs as the water escapes the blood vessels because there is not enough protein in the blood vessels to hold it in place. (For the scientists, water needs the osmotic draw of protein to stay in the blood vessel; otherwise, it escapes to create osmotic equilibrium.)

Lastly, injuries like infections, arthritis, gout, or a sprained ankle result in edema as the body sends its best weapons to heal itself. It sends chemicals to treat infections, to build a wall around an infection (abscess), thereby preventing spread to other parts of the body, to remove harmful byproducts like crystals, and to heal injured tissues. Swollen areas of your body should never be red. That is a reason to call your doctor immediately.

When patients have edema, they usually notice swelling or puffiness of the skin, which then appears stretched. Edema near joints, will make joints feel stiff and achy. To see if you have edema, push on your skin for five seconds over the shinbone and then let go. Edema will usually leave a temporary dent (pitting edema). Edema from injury, though, usually doesn't leave dents.

What You Can Do for Yourself

- Elevate your legs, ideally above the heart, for as much of the day and night as you can. Perhaps use a recliner during the day and put your legs on a pillow at night.
- When your legs are dangling, wear support or compression stockings. Yes, they can be very difficult to put on. If someone is helping you, have them sit next to you and pull on the stockings, rather than sit across from you and try to push them on. Consider stockings with zippers to make them easier to put on. Many of my patients like using Circaid® compression stockings and feel they are worth the investment. If they are too tight or not tight enough, ask for a different level of pressure.
- Exercise your legs, ankles, and feet.
- Don't sit for prolonged periods of time.
- Consume a low-salt diet.
- Ask your doctor how much water you should drink, and then keep track of your daily intake of fluids. Most people need to drink more water . . . but that may not be the case if you have congestive heart failure, liver disease, or kidney failure; then you need to drink much less.

- Gently massage your legs. This helps push the fluid back into the blood vessels and allows your kidneys to urinate out the excess fluid.
- Baths can help too but should only be used if the skin is intact and you can safely get in and out of the bathtub. Just the gentle pressure from the bathwater will help push fluid back into the blood vessels!

What Your Doctor Can Do

- Let you know how much water you should be drinking per day.
- Your doctor should review your medications to see if any of them cause edema and adjust doses whenever possible.
- Your doctor should rule out dangerous causes of edema, like blood clots (deep venous thrombosis) and liver, kidney, or heart failure.
- Sometimes, doctors will provide water pills like furosemide (Lasix®), but I find that things you can do for yourself are more effective and have fewer side effects.

You Control the Outcome

This is another example where you have more power to affect the outcome than your doctor does. Certainly, you need your doctor to ensure that nothing dangerous or life-threatening is causing the problem. Once those things are ruled out, the treatment is in your hands. A few lifestyle modifications can make a world of difference in terms of comfort and your ability to move around.

I can tell you what happens if edema goes untreated. Imagine that you have very swollen legs, and you continue to eat a high-salt, fast-food diet every day and avoid elevating your legs except when lying flat in bed at night. You don't exercise but spend countless consecutive hours on the couch watching television and drinking liters of soda. Eventually, you will require periodic hospitalizations, when your legs get so swollen that they leaked fluid right through the skin! These porous areas then get infected with staph and strep bacteria that normally live peacefully and harmlessly on your skin. Now these infections require two weeks of IV antibiotics to treat and continue to recur. Pretty soon, you are falling out of bed because your legs are so heavy that you can no longer move without a safety risk . . . and the downward spiral continues.

I much prefer to tell you the story of ninety-four-year-old Mildred with chronic swelling in her ankles, who just came back from a trip to Hawaii. She took the trip by herself for no special reason other than she thought she deserved it. She reported that she was sure to bring her compression stockings on the flight to control the swelling and was careful to eat a low-salt diet and keep up her walking while traveling. She reported that the airline even let her bring her CPAP machine (for sleep apnea) as a carry-on without a problem.

Then there is eighty-one-year-old Harry, who did everything I suggested to reduce the swelling in his legs and ankles so that he could dance comfortably with his wife at their sixtieth wedding anniversary. You know, the next week, he brought me a picture of them dancing AND a picture of his ankles in his fancy dancing shoes!

Mildred and Harry felt so empowered by their decisions and their actions. They were living their best lives. Regardless of the outcome, they knew that they were in charge of their senior years and that their senior years were not in charge of them.

CHAPTER SIXTEEN
FOOT CARE: SUPPORT YOUR FOUNDATION

Your Structural Foundation

Do you remember the kid's song "Head, Shoulders, Knees, and Toes"? I must not forget the body's structural foundation. It's both the feet and toes! You may wonder why your doctor is always taking off your shoes and socks to look at your feet. First of all, some of you have trouble seeing the bottoms of your feet, and somebody has to look at them. Secondly, they tell doctors a lot of information about your circulation, your body's ability to heal itself, how well you can fight infections, the progression of your chronic diseases, and they help your doctor anticipate future problems. Lastly, many patients struggle with common foot problems.

Willard had developed back pain which he attributed to his new limp. His left lower back and buttock hurt, and he explained that he "just can't walk right anymore." When I watched him walk into the exam room, out of the corner of my eye, I noticed that he was walking on the outside of his left foot. With a flick of my wrist, off came his shoes and socks. He had a huge corn on the ball of his foot. A little frozen spray to numb the area and a quick wielding of a skilled hand and a knife (don't try this at home), and I removed a large corn. Not a single drop of blood was lost, and he left the office walking on the soles of both feet, hopeful that his back would heal quickly!

Changes with Age

Over time, the foot naturally gets wider. The arch drops, and the soft tissues of the foot stretch. Some women notice this during pregnancy, while others notice it if they gain weight for other reasons. Regardless, everyone's feet will widen. So don't hesitate to buy wider shoes if needed as it will save you from other problems, such as corns, blisters, and calluses. You may also notice that while you may be gaining weight in unwanted places, you are losing the cushioning fat pads under the ball of your foot and heel. This can lead to pain if your shoes do not have adequate soles. Consider a shoe with a thicker, softer sole or orthotics to help compensate for these changes.

Common Foot Disorders

Here are my thoughts on some of the other common foot problems that we see:

Flat Feet

Did you know that injuries, diabetes, obesity, and even high blood pressure all cause flat feet? When tendons that support your arch get weak or damaged, you lose the arch in your foot.

What You Can Do for Yourself

- Orthotics are the way to go to avoid foot, ankle, knee, and back pain . . . oh, and future arthritis! You can either buy them over the counter or go to a podiatrist.

What Your Doctor Can Do

- Confirm the diagnosis.
- Order custom orthotics.

Plantar Fasciitis

This is the most common foot complaint. When you stand up, usually from bed in the morning or after sitting for a long time, it feels like something is being torn off of your heel. The plantar fascia runs the length of your foot, supporting the arch, but if it gets tight and angry, it feels like it is about to be ripped off of your heel right where the heel meets the arch of the foot. Plantar fasciitis can also cause stiffness. It is caused by repetitive injury from jogging or walking or from being immobilized in a boot or cast. People with high arches and who are overweight are more likely to suffer from this injury.

What You Can Do for Yourself

- Unless you have had it before, go to your doctor to get the diagnosis confirmed.
- Treat your symptoms with rest, ice, acetaminophen (Tylenol®), ibuprofen (Motrin®), or naproxen (Aleve®). Check with your doctor before taking ibuprofen or naproxen.
- Stretch your calf muscle.
- Roll the bottom of your foot over a tennis ball or frozen ball!
- Wear prefabricated silicone heel inserts.
- Until fully healed, only wear athletic shoes with good arch support . . . not even slippers or being barefoot are allowed! While it may seem strange, that means putting on your sneakers before getting out of bed.

What Your Doctor Can Do

- Confirm the diagnosis.
- Refer you to physical therapy or review exercises with you.
- Show you how to tape your foot.
- Offer steroid injections if the above treatments don't work.
- Other options include iontophoresis, short-leg walking cast, or, rarely, surgery.
- Treatments tried without proven success include: extracorporeal shockwave therapy, autologous whole-blood or platelet-rich plasma injections, botulinum toxin injections, topical wheatgrass cream, radiotherapy, cryosurgery, low-level laser therapy, electric dry needling, and micronized dehydrated human amnion injection.

Morton's Neuromas

Up to 33 percent of people will get these in their lifetime. These occur when the nerve sheath between your third and fourth toe becomes inflamed. Patients complain of pain in the front part of their foot or that it feels like they are walking on a rock. This is more common in people who wear high-heeled shoes or shoes with a tight toe box.

What You Can Do for Yourself

- Wear shoes with a broad toe space and softer soles.
- Get foot massages (or just pretend you have a neuroma and get foot massages anyway!).

What Your Doctor Can Do

- Confirm the diagnosis.
- Create a metatarsal support, bar, or padding for your shoe.
- Provide exercises to strengthen the foot muscles.
- Offer glucocorticoid shots, or alcohol and radiofrequency ablation, or, rarely, surgery.

Cracked Skin

With age, people become more dehydrated, and dry weather certainly doesn't help. The skin also loses oil and elastin, making it stiffer and more likely to crack (the same applies to the cracks in your fingers).

What You Can Do for Yourself

- Be sure to apply moisturizing lotion to your feet every day.
- Keratolytics (like CeraVe® SA cream) can be used to remove rough skin.
- Sand down the thick areas with a pumice stone.
- If you are diabetic or have neuropathy, please let a podiatrist take care of your feet rather than trying to do it yourself.
- If your feet are ever swollen or red, see your doctor.

What Your Doctor Can Do

- Recommend specific lotions.
- Safely cut away thick patches of skin.
- Treat and prevent infections.

Ingrown Toenails

This occurs when the side of the nail grows into the skin, causing pain, swelling, and, often, infection. This can be avoided by not cutting your toenails too short and wearing wider-toed shoes.

What You Can Do for Yourself

- Don't cut your toenails too short.
- If you can pull the corner of the nail above the skin, it will likely resolve on its own.
- However, if you are diabetic or it is red and infected, see your doctor.

What Your Doctor Can Do

- Cut your toenails safely and to the appropriate length.
- Gently lift the corners of your toenails to allow ingrown nails to heal. They often put some cotton under the corner as well.
- Treat and prevent infection.

Ulcers

Foot ulcers are more common in people who have neuropathy and can't feel the bottoms of their feet. They may get a small pebble in their shoe or even the seam of a sock may cause an unnoticed break in the skin, leading to an ulcer. The smallest blister can turn into a big infection that spreads deep into the bone, leading to weeks of IV antibiotics and, sometimes, amputations.

What You Can Do for Yourself

- If you have numbness or abnormal sensations in your feet, wear closed shoes to avoid getting debris in your shoes.

- If you have numbness or abnormal sensations in your feet, check your feet for injury every day and have a doctor check your feet three to four times a year.
- If you are diabetic and you find an open sore or ulcer, see your doctor.
- If you are not a diabetic and you find an open sore or ulcer, wash it out with water and then make sure it heals within a week. If you notice redness, swelling, white (pus) drainage, or it smells, that is also when you should seek medical attention.

What Your Doctor Can Do

- Ensure that your wound heals properly.
- Treat and prevent infection.

Bunions

First, check out your parents' feet. Bunions are usually inherited. If you got "bunion" genes, you might start to notice your big toe starting to turn in towards the little toes and a lump appearing where the big toe meets the foot.

What You Can Do for Yourself

- Avoid tight, narrow shoes and high heels.
- Wear loose shoes.
- Place special pads over the bunions.
- When the bunions hurt or are inflamed, ice is the best treatment. Acetaminophen (Tylenol®), ibuprofen (Motrin®), or naproxen (Aleve®) help too. Check with your doctor before taking ibuprofen or naproxen.
- If that doesn't help, go to your doctor.

What Your Doctor Can Do

- Make you orthotics.
- Offer you splinting options and exercises.
- Discuss surgical correction.

Fungal Infections

Cracks in the skin and a weaker immune system that naturally comes with age increase one's risk for fungal infections. With fungal infections, the sole of the foot scales and then itches. Without treatment, the infection can spread to the toenails, where it is much harder to treat.

What You Can Do for Yourself

- Try over-the-counter antifungal creams or sprays, but if they don't work quickly and resolve the problem 100 percent, then go to your doctor.
- Please don't put steroid cream on these rashes, as it will worsen the infection.

What Your Doctor Can Do

- Confirm the diagnosis.
- Provide stronger treatment options and ideally prevent the nails from getting infected.

Corns and Calluses

While they are just thickening of the skin, corns and calluses can cause considerable pain, discomfort, and disability. If they cause you to walk differently, it can cause pain in other joints and your back, too! Those with hammertoes can even get corns and calluses on the tops of their toes. While there are several over-the-counter products for corns and calluses, I find that what doctors, including podiatrists, have to offer works better and quicker. And they can help you prevent recurrent corns and calluses.

What You Can Do for Yourself

- Let your doctor just take care of it. Otherwise, you will be fighting with the over-the-counter products for months.

What Your Doctor Can Do

- Magically make them go away!
- And try to prevent recurrences.

CHAPTER SIXTEEN

Foot Care

In our community, there are nurses that will go to people's homes and assist with toenail trimming. And podiatrists offer in-office nail trimming, as this can become more difficult as nails thicken with age.

When my new spouse and I joined homes, we joyfully unpacked box after box. At one point, I discovered a Dremel and shouted, "I'm so glad we have a Dremel!"

"Why?" echoed from another basement closet.

"Because now when I get old, I can trim my old lady toenails!"

Twenty-plus years ago, when I worked in rural America taking care of geriatric patients, I often used a Dremel to sand down thick toenails. It took time and made a lot of dust, but it worked beautifully. (If you are diabetic or can't feel your feet, don't try this at home.)

We all need a stable foundation. Don't forget to clean the feet at least weekly with a good sudsy soak and gently scrub with a washcloth, trim the nails regularly, and see a podiatrist if needed. It is important to stay upright and to move for as long as possible so you can be off to the next adventure!

CHAPTER SEVENTEEN
MEDICATION DOSING: START LOW AND GO SLOW

It's Just a Beer

Imagine this. You decide to take your twenty-two-year-old grandson to see his favorite baseball team. At the start of the first inning, he generously runs to the concession stand and brings back a strong craft beer for each of you to enjoy. Together, you sit with smiles on your faces as you share time with your grandson, and you each drink a beer. The home team scores a run. You are feeling warm and happy. Then, your grandson wants a second beer. Not to be outdone by your grandson, you acquiesce and have a second. You are now drunk, and he barely notices a difference in himself as he cheers for his team, the Colorado Rockies. The bases are now loaded . . . and so are you.

Fast forward twelve hours. Your grandson gets woken up by his college roommates who are making noise. He jumps in the shower, grabs a quick breakfast, and heads off to class. The only thing on his mind is making it to class on time. You, on the other hand, have a list of regrets. You didn't sleep well at all compared to the modest sleep you usually get. Your stomach didn't tolerate the alcohol at all, and you are feeling the remnants of last night's heartburn. As you lay in bed with a headache, you chuckle, remembering how many beers you were able to drink when you were a twenty-two-year-old and wonder what has changed. Do the craft beers have more alcohol than beers you used to drink?

CHAPTER SEVENTEEN

Aging Bodies React Differently to Chemicals

As the body gets older, there are shifts in the amount of water, fat, and protein in one's body. This affects how chemicals, like alcohol and medications, impact the body. As one ages, the amount of water in our body goes down, leaving the body in a chronic state of dehydration. For most people, the percentage of fat tends to go up, and with muscle loss, the amount of protein goes down. Good news. These are not all inevitable. Muscle loss with age is known as sarcopenia and is preventable with exercise and a healthy diet.

Let's discuss body water first. Babies are 78 percent water, and by age one, they are 68 percent water. By middle age, there is a fair amount of variability between individuals, but men are approximately 60 percent water and women 55 percent. With age, this can drop to 50 percent for males and 45 percent for females. We go from 78 percent water down to as low as 45 percent!

Now, let's take a look at the alcohol example. What happens if you pour a pint of beer into bucket A that contains sixty cups of water versus bucket B that contains fifty cups? The concentration of beer in bucket B is much higher, and if you were to drink from both buckets, the beer in bucket B would seem stronger. The same is true for the human body. As the body ages and has less water in it, alcohol floats around the bloodstream at a higher concentration, causing you to get drunk on less beer. Likewise, medications of the same dose float around the body at higher concentrations and are more potent. This also explains why older people experience more side effects from medications. This is true for all medications that dissolve in water. These medications need to be dosed at a lower amount as you age. Atenolol (Tenormin®) is an example of a water-soluble heart medication that is sometimes used for blood pressure. Sometimes, patients will want to know why their doctors are lowering the dose of their medications as they get older or why they don't need as much blood pressure medication, and this is why.

Medications are a bit like baking ingredients. Some mix better in water, and some mix more readily with oils. Some medications prefer to attach themselves to fat molecules rather than mix with all of the water in your body. As you age and acquire more fat, these medications stay in your system for longer periods of time. These medications need to be dosed farther apart as you age, say every six hours instead of every four. One example of a medication that binds to fat is lorazepam (Ativan®), a medication for anxiety. One dose will stay in your body for an unpredictably long period of time, depending on how much body fat you have. There are some medications, like amiodarone, that if you get one dose, because it has such a long half-life, it may be in your body for the rest of your life.

Lastly, some medications bind to protein. When you take medication that binds to protein, some of the medication exists in the body partially bound to protein while the rest floats free in your system in its active form. If you have less protein in your body for medication to bind to, then there will be more active medication available floating free. These medications need to be dosed at a lower amount as you age. Warfarin (Coumadin®), which is a blood thinner, binds to proteins. As you get older or lose muscle mass during an illness or a sedentary period, your usual dose will result in a more potent response, thinning your blood too much. Blood testing of your PT/INR will allow you and your doctor to adjust the dose to ensure that the active form of this medication floating free is at the proper level and that your blood is neither too thin nor too thick.

Medication Dosing Will Change

Your doctor and pharmacist will know which medications fall into which categories, so don't be surprised if medication doses get adjusted as you age. Also, don't be surprised if your doctor prefers to start at a low dose and slowly titrate up new medications. Now you will understand why it is important with medicine to start low and go slow! This requires extra patience awaiting medication results, but it is well worth the wait to avoid unpleasant and even dangerous side effects.

Here are a few other random things that you might find interesting about how your body metabolizes medications as you age. It takes longer for your gastrointestinal tract to absorb many medications. Your stomach also becomes less acidic, making it more difficult for some medications to be absorbed. Lastly, the liver and kidneys clear medication from the body more slowly, so medication effects and their side effects tend to hang around for longer periods of time. Almost all antibiotics are given at a lower dose as you age, as well as allopurinol for gout, ranitidine for heartburn, gabapentin for nerve pain, and more. More reasons to start with lower doses at wider time intervals. The motto is start low and go slow!

Proceed with More Caution

You likely remember Aesop's fable of "The Tortoise and the Hare" from your childhood. If not, I won't give the specific details away. Feel free to read it to your grandchildren or other children in your life. It teaches us that there is value in going slow. Slow teaches us patience and hones acceptance and gratitude. Going slow allows for small mistakes rather than large mistakes that are hard to recover from. Slow limits injury and damage. Slow builds resilience and strength. Have you tried weightlifting slow rather than fast? If you have, then you can appreciate the results. Slow allows for contemplation and thought and to feel emotions more deeply. Slow brings greater clarity. Don't be afraid of slow. With slow comes gifts. Gifts that your doctors have already come to realize.

As you can tell from the prior chapters, medications are only a small portion of a patient's treatment plan. No pill will serve as the instant cure. You and your doctors can work on other modalities of treatment, like topical medications with fewer side effects, physical therapy, massage, diet, exercise, acupuncture, meditation, and so on, if you are waiting for medications to take full effect and be maximized. There are so many avenues to feeling better, living better, and experiencing life at its best. Consider them all.

CHAPTER EIGHTEEN
SENSORY LOSS: "IT HELPS TO BE A LITTLE DEAF"

The Senses Fade

Ruth Bader Ginsburg passed on much wisdom in her lifetime. One piece of wisdom she reportedly got from her mother-in-law was that "in every good marriage, it helps to be a little deaf." I would imagine that there are times that being a little blind is to one's advantage as well. But what if hearing loss is not a choice but rather comes with time and years of hard work? Some people lose their vision in one eye or both. At its worst, some are robbed of both sight and hearing.

There is one thing that I haven't quite figured out. Most of my patients who have become hearing-impaired as they age choose not to wear their hearing aids. Do hearing aids make them feel old? Are the hearing aids physically uncomfortable? Do they amplify unpleasant sounds or too much background noise? Are the devices too complicated? Are they too ugly? Do they prefer not to hear what is happening around them? Is it too exhausting and overstimulating to struggle to hear and easier just to not hear at all? Have they lost their hearing aids, and are they too expensive to replace (or buy in the first place)? What I see is the isolation and depression that follows as one slowly loses their hearing and becomes disconnected from the world around them. Clearly, I lack full understanding of this frequent choice that frustrates everyone around the hearing impaired and leads to their overall functional decline.

I don't see the same with vision impairment. Lots of people wear glasses every day and don't think twice about it unless there is a smudge or raindrops on the lenses. Most people are willing to throw on a pair of glasses without a blink of an eye to read fine print. In fact, many people leave several pairs of "readers" throughout their homes so as to have them readily accessible when needed. Clearly, their utility is more than a fashion statement; otherwise, they would wear them all the time.

Hearing Loss

All of our senses diminish with age, but most people don't feel as limited if their sense of taste decreases as they do if they experience hearing loss or vision loss. Age-related hearing loss is called presbycusis. It is one of the most common conditions affecting older adults, with nearly half of seventy-five-year-olds experiencing significant hearing loss. Usually, both ears are affected, almost equally, and it occurs so gradually over time that often it goes unnoticed until someone subtly or not so subtly points it out. The innocent five-year-old asks, "Grandma, why is your television so loud?" or your son rudely says, "Ma! You are deaf as a doornail. When are you going to get hearing aids?"

Older people experience three types of hearing loss. In order to understand how the ear becomes damaged with time, it helps to understand how the ear works. Sounds enter the ear through the ear canal. In the outer ear, sound waves are amplified and strike the eardrum (tympanic membrane). The eardrum vibrates, moving the three inner ear bones—the malleus, incus, and stapes—that, like a chain reaction, activate the inner ear. When the stapes knocks on the base of the cochlea in the inner ear, fluid in the cochlea ripples through the ear, bending the hair cells that line the inside of the canals. The moving hair cells translate each vibration into an electrical signal that the brain can interpret as a sound that we recognize and can understand (see Figure 18.1).

Noise-induced hearing loss is caused by years of exposure to loud and/or persistent sounds. These sounds damage and break off the hair cells, and once they are damaged, they do not get repaired or grow back. Damage to the nerves of the ears that transmit and read the electrical signals in the brain can be caused by years of disease such as high blood pressure,

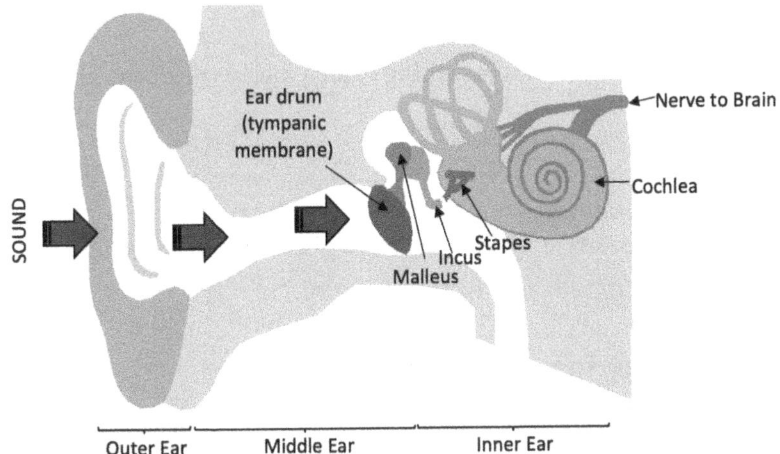

Figure 18.1. Anatomy of the entire ear. This figure demonstrates how sound enters the ear and is communicated to the brain.

diabetes, and medications. Lastly, many people produce ear wax, which can block soundwaves from entering the outer ear and reaching the eardrum unobstructed.

What You Can Do for Yourself

- The best way to prevent hearing loss is to wear ear protection when working with loud noises or persistent noises. Please do this even if you have already lost hearing.
- Work with your doctor to manage your chronic illnesses.
- Ask your doctor if your ears need to be cleaned of wax.
- Everyone who is concerned that their hearing is diminished should get their hearing checked by an audiologist.
- At age sixty-five, regardless of how well you think you hear, you should have your hearing checked and then periodically after that, depending on the results. If you need a hearing aid, the audiologist can send you in the proper direction. For more complex hearing problems, you may be referred to an otolaryngologist, also known as an ears, nose, and throat (ENT) doctor.

What Your Doctor Can Do

- Diagnose and treat underlying health problems that may contribute to hearing loss.
- Check your ears for wax and clean wax out of your ear.
- Refer you for a hearing test or to an otolaryngologist, also known as an ears, nose, and throat (ENT) doctor.
- Refer you to a speech and language pathologist or occupational therapist to help you adapt to life with impaired hearing.

Treatment for Hearing Loss

The most common treatment for hearing loss is hearing aids because they make sounds louder. They come in many styles, including behind the ear, mini behind the eye, in the ear, in the canal, and completely-in-the-canal. People often need to try multiple styles to find the one that is most comfortable. Once you get a hearing aid, be sure that you know how to put it in, take it out, clean it, adjust the volume, and change the batteries. Smartphones now have apps that connect to hearing aids so that cell phones can be amplified through hearing aids. There are also amplifier boxes for people who cannot afford to wear hearing aids. You may also want to check out the free app Ava that types out spoken words, so those hard of hearing can follow conversations. I use it all the time with patients, especially when we have to wear face masks. If these don't work, there are more complex devices and language boards that can be used for communication. Your audiologist and speech and language pathologist will have more options, but what I covered works for most people.

Currently, genetic risk factors for hearing loss are being studied as well as the potential for regrowing hair cells or using gene therapy to restore hearing. There is also research being done to improve upon the current hearing aid devices.

Vision Loss

One universal age-related vision challenge is called presbyopia. Starting in your forties, the lens of the eye becomes less flexible, making it more difficult to focus on close objects. By fifty years old, there is a wish for the arms to be six inches longer so you can read fine print. Sometimes people start developing headaches or tired eyes while reading. This is correctable with over-the-counter readers for most people. If your left and right eyes need different prescriptions, you may need custom lenses to be measured by an optometrist and made by an optician.

Fortunately, I wear glasses all of the time. The low humidity in Colorado (often less than 10 percent) makes it difficult to wear contacts due to dry eyes, and given my work, I appreciate the extra eye protection. When the doctor said I needed "readers," also known as reading glasses, I was able to hide them in my regular everyday lenses, providing just the slightest illusion that I might still be a young adult! Of course, this is a joke, which you might not realize unless you knew me. My hair has turned gray, and I've chosen to fully embrace it. The truth is, I'm enjoying getting older.

The remaining eye conditions that affect older people do so more variably. Not everyone is affected, and some people have minimal symptoms while others are seriously disabled by them.

Common Eye Problems in the Elderly

The eye is normally filled with a very thick liquid substance like honey (vitreous). As you age, the consistency thins in sections, causing areas that are still the thickness of honey to clump together. These clumps cause shadows that float across one's vision and are perceived as small dark shapes, called floaters. They can look like spots, threads, wavy lines, or cobwebs. Most floaters eventually float to the side and out of the way of your central vision.

The proteins in the lens of the eye behave a lot like the vitreous in the eye. They break down with time and clump together, clouding vision. By age eighty, half of Americans have had or need cataract surgery. Diseases like diabetes, high blood pressure (hypertension), obesity, and the use of steroids, alcohol, and tobacco can accelerate the development of cataracts. Patients with cataracts often experience cloudy, blurred, or dim vision, difficulty seeing at night, sensitivity to light, halos around lights, and fading color intensity.

As people are more dehydrated in general with age, they make fewer tears, and their eyes get drier. Without tears, eyes become inflamed, and the cornea can get damaged, affecting vision. Think of it this way: The cornea is like the window of the eye. If the window gets dry, the eyelids are more likely to scratch the window and blur the view through the window. People with dry eyes are bothered by stinging, burning, scratchy eyes; stringy eye mucus; sensitivity to light; red eyes; and a sensation that something is in their eyes. People will also report blurred vision and eye fatigue, with an inability to wear contacts. (And I blame it all on the lack of humidity in the air!)

Glaucoma is the leading cause of blindness in people over sixty, but it is treatable. The problem is that without regular eye exams, it often goes unnoticed. It is caused by elevated pressure in the eye that puts pressure on and damages the optic nerve. Vision loss begins in the peripheral vision and is painless. It often goes unnoticed until much vision is lost and the damage reaches the central area of vision. People with very poor vision, diabetes, high blood pressure, heart disease, who take steroid medications, or have family members with glaucoma are more likely to get it. If you have glaucoma, let your doctors know so that they resist giving you eye drops with steroids because steroids increase eye pressure.

Macular degeneration affects ten million aging Americans, and that is more than cataracts and glaucoma combined. The retina is the portion of the eye that lines the inside of the eyeball, and it records images that are sent via the optic nerve to the brain to be interpreted. Macular degeneration causes deterioration of the retina, but unlike glaucoma that affects the peripheral vision, macular degeneration affects your most valuable central

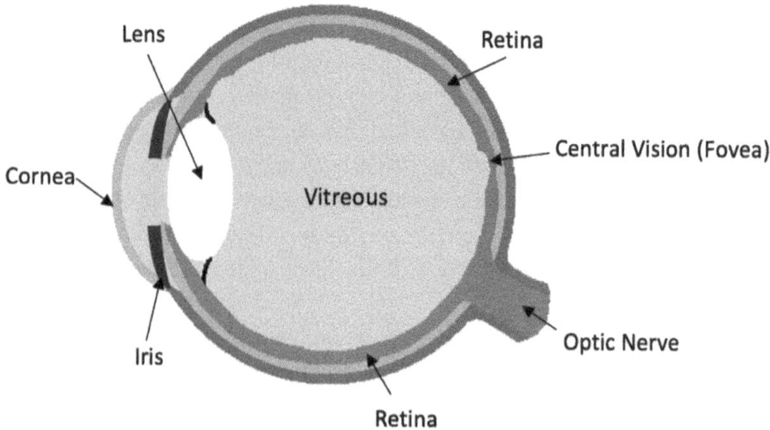

Figure 18.2. Anatomy of the eye.

vision that you need to focus on books and other objects, the television, landscapes, faces . . . everything. Imagine sticking a nickel-sized piece of wax paper to the center of each lens of your glasses. Now put on your glasses and try to see. That is what it is like to have macular degeneration. Smoking tobacco doubles your risk of this disease. Caucasians and people with a family history are also at a higher risk.

What You Can Do for Yourself

- Sunglasses go a long way in protecting one's eyes (and prevent wrinkles! See Chapter 4). And they can be worn in the winter as well as the summer. Some older people can develop pterygiums from the sun, which are pink triangles of tissue that grow over the cornea. They are usually harmless and don't affect vision, but they can bother people for cosmetic reasons. Pterygiums can be prevented by wearing sunglasses.
- Choose a healthy diet full of omega-3s, carotenoids, lutein, zeaxanthin, and zinc!
- Talk to your doctor about how best to quit tobacco and alcohol.
- Physical activity . . . yes, it does seem to help everything.
- Put a bright light on the subject to help overcome early declines in vision. When the print at work is too small, or the splinter I'm removing from someone's hand is too blurry, I just need to turn up the light . . . and to wear my glasses.
- Can you enlarge the font or buy print that is larger?
- Do you have a magnifying glass with a light at the ready for when you have vision challenges reading small print?
- Get your eyes examined at least every one to two years to look for eye disease and to adjust prescriptions in your glasses and contacts. Ask about lens filters to help you see better in different environments.
- If your eyes are dry, stay hydrated and talk to your doctor about lubricating drops, higher-viscosity artificial tear gels, and ointments. Avoid wind, drafts, and, when needed, humidify your environment. Some eyeglass stores sell "moisture chamber glasses" to create a physical barrier around the eye to preserve the humidity around the eye. (Welcome to the Southwest!)

- If you have glaucoma, the best thing you can do for yourself is to take your eye drops regularly and get your eye pressure checked as recommended.
- For macular degeneration, there are two types:
    - Dry type: Ask your doctor about oral antioxidant vitamins like PreserVisionAREDS 2 and statin therapy.
    - Wet type: Ask your doctor about oral antioxidant vitamins like PreserVisionAREDS 2.
- I love all types of therapy. And there is occupational therapy for everything including vision loss. If you have lost vision, ask. It will change your life! They can teach you how to adapt to your new level of ability.
- If you have a sudden change in vision, call your doctor or go to the emergency room immediately. If vision is to be recovered, it must be recovered quickly, and the doctors need to make sure that you aren't having a stroke.

What Your Doctor Can Do

- Examine your eyes to look for any eye diseases or age-related changes.
- Be available to evaluate all sudden loss of vision.
- If your eyes are dry, your doctor may perform a procedure called punctal occlusion to block the tear drain so that the tears stay in the eye longer. It's like plugging the drain in your bathroom sink. They may also recommend prescription medications to stimulate tears, vitamins, large specially fitted contact lenses, acupuncture, or surgery to correct eyelid abnormalities or damage to the cornea. New types of eye drops—diquafosol and rebamipide—are being investigated.
- If you have glaucoma, your doctor can provide prescription eye drops, laser treatment, and surgeries that can help slow down the progression of glaucoma.
- If you have cataracts, surgery to replace cataracts is well tolerated at all ages.
- For macular degeneration, there are two types:

  - Dry type: Your doctor can recommend oral antioxidant vitamins, zinc, and statin therapy. Stem cells are being studied. Laser therapy was shown to cause more harm than benefit. At some point, doctors may offer stem cell treatment.
  - Wet type: Your doctor can recommend an oral antioxidant and provide intraocular injections called vascular endothelial growth factor inhibitors. Photodynamic therapy and thermal laser photocoagulation have become less popular with the introduction of newer therapeutic agents, with fewer side effects and greater efficacy. These therapies in combination are currently being studied. Surgeries have had mixed results, and some are still considered experimental.
- Order occupational therapy!

Hope through Progress

What I see is how hearing aids have changed over the years. The first hearing aids consisted of large animal horns placed in each ear to amplify sound. In the 1950s, hearing aids were made like transistor radios. By the late twentieth century, they were small enough to clip to the ear. By the end of the twentieth century, hearing aids had become small digital devices that hung over the ear or were small enough to fit in the ear canal itself. They are more comfortable, have become better at blocking out background noise, the batteries last longer, and they are now programmable. They have certainly come a long way from putting a ten-inch animal horn up to your ear. And I expect progress to continue! Technology moves fast. With an aging population and a growing market, I anticipate that assistive devices will continue to improve in leaps and bounds. Perhaps someday they will be even better than our own ears!

What I also remember are the thick, truly glass eyeglass lenses that my dad used to wear. They were about five pounds and left huge crater-like dents in his nose and behind his ears. Now his eyeglass lenses are plastic and ground down to featherweight, become tinted in the sun, resist glare, and are scratch resistant, not to mention they allow him to see at all distances without the bifocal line. Are his eyes any better? No. Technology is!

So, despite being forty years older, he sees better than when he was in his thirties. No matter where you are in life today, there is hope that tomorrow will afford something new, exciting, different, and better. Until then, there are things you can do to launch yourself forward.

CHAPTER NINETEEN

MILD COGNITIVE IMPAIRMENT AND DEMENTIA: IT'S JUST A SENIOR MOMENT . . . RIGHT?

Where Did It Go?

A week went by where I kept losing my keys. One Saturday afternoon, I looked all over the house for those darn keys. They weren't in their usual location in the house where I normally put my keys. They weren't in my work bag or in my coat pocket. I hadn't dropped them in the closet. They weren't in the pocket of the pants that I had worn the day before. The hamper was turned upside down without a single jingle. I checked the kitchen counters. The path from the garage to the house is short and cement. It was bare. With generosity of heart, my spouse began looking with me. The garbage was a mess but keyless. The drawers, once clean, became tumultuously disappointing. "It's just a senior moment . . . right?" I joked. Finally, I relinquished myself of that frantic energy of searching for something lost and agreed to let my spouse drive us to the store. As we got near her car, she pulled MY keys from HER jacket pocket. Did I mention that I'm the younger spouse? Got to run . . .

If you have lost your keys recently, don't panic. Everyone loses their keys. That is not a sign of dementia. Dementia is when you forget what keys are for!

Forgetfulness is a normal part of aging, and as we age, it takes longer to learn new things. Some of our brain cells die each year, causing our brains to shrink, but we have billions of cells in reserve so that we can continue to function with day-to-day activities. By age seventy, about 8 percent of people will have mild cognitive impairment, and by age eighty-five, 25 percent will have it. Of people over eighty-five, 16 percent develop dementia.

Normal versus Disease

What is the difference between normal aging and more serious trouble like mild cognitive impairment or dementia? If you are starting to ask the same questions over and over again, getting lost in familiar places, having trouble following instructions, struggling to find words, or becoming confused with time, people, and places, then it is time to talk to your doctor. Your doctor can perform an extensive history to determine the nature of your specific deficits, review your medical problems, consider the medications you are taking, including supplements, and complete a physical exam, including a thorough neurological exam. The doctor may want to get information from a close relative or friend to see how they perceive your functioning.

Then your doctor will ask you to complete a cognitive test, either the mini-mental status exam (MMSE), the Montreal Cognitive Assessment (MoCA), or the Saint Louis University Mental Status (SLUMS). Your score on these exams is relative to your education, age, and functional ability. Depending on your performance, your doctor may recommend lab tests like a vitamin B12 level, thyroid tests, a depression screen, more comprehensive neuropsychiatric testing, and/or an MRI or CT scan. Patients with a low B12 level can experience a decline in memory, understanding, and judgment. Thyroid disease can present with forgetfulness. Depression or distracting anxiety can present with the same symptoms as dementia, which is why it is sometimes referred to as pseudodementia. Structural abnormalities in the brain can push on structures that result in deficits similar to dementia. If the patient is a heavy drinker of alcohol, a vitamin B1 level should be checked to ensure that the symptoms are not caused by thiamine deficiency.

Risk factors for mild cognitive impairment are advancing age, family history of Alzheimer's or other forms of dementia, and cardiovascular disease like strokes (cerebrovascular accidents), heart attacks (myocardial infarctions), and high cholesterol (hyperlipidemia).

Your doctor may tell you that you are completely normal and that your experiences are consistent with others your age. This may result in mixed emotions of relief that you don't have dementia and frustration that your brain isn't working like a twenty-year-old anymore. How hard will it be to accept that there is no quick fix?

Mild Cognitive Impairment

If you are diagnosed with mild cognitive impairment (MCI), you are likely experiencing symptoms on a more consistent basis than your similarly aged friends whose brains are aging normally. Compared to them, if you have an amnestic mild cognitive impairment, you will forget things more often. This includes names, appointments, and social events but have preserved general cognitive function. Some patients experience loss in multiple domains with or without forgetfulness (amnestic MCI versus non-amnestic MCI). They may also lose their train of thought and/or have more trouble following conversations. They may misplace things more than they did a decade prior. They may feel overwhelmed with making decisions, planning, and following instructions and take longer to navigate previously familiar environments. It is not uncommon for patients with mild cognitive impairment to become a bit more impulsive, begin to demonstrate poor judgment, and experience depression, irritability, anxiety, and even apathy. While these symptoms are all noticeable to close family members, they still do not significantly impact daily functioning. They are bumps in the road and obstacles that are surmountable. Patients often develop techniques to overcome their deficits and continue to function in the world. Rarely do the general public or friends notice. Unlike dementia, memory deficits with mild cognitive impairment can remain stable for years, without decline. To relieve anxiety, let me say that again: memory deficits with mild cognitive impairment can remain stable for years, without decline.

Dementia

Of patients with MCI, 10 percent per year progress to dementia. The term dementia encompasses many diseases that cause loss of memory, language, problem-solving skills, and critical thinking that are severe enough to interfere with daily living despite attempts to compensate for one's deficits. Neuropsychiatric testing of patients with MCI can indicate who is more likely to develop dementia, as can a slow gait, loss of the sense of smell, APOE epsilon 4 genotype, cerebrovascular disease, certain biomarkers in the fluid around the brain and spinal cord (tau or tau protein phosphorylated at Tau-181 and lower levels of amyloid beta 42 [Aß42] peptide, a low ratio of Aß42 to Aß40 levels, and a low ratio of Aß42 to tau levels), and structural abnormalities on a brain MRI. There are ongoing studies on the usefulness of blood tests (plasma biomarkers) and newer imaging tests (FDG-PET and functional MRI, amyloid PET, and Tau PET) for predicting dementia.

The general term dementia includes many diseases, such as Alzheimer's dementia, vascular dementia, Lewy body dementia, Parkinson's dementia, frontotemporal dementia, Creutzfeldt-Jakob disease, normal pressure hydrocephalus, and Wernicke-Korsakoff syndrome. Thus, Alzheimer's is a type of dementia. Patients can also have more than one type of dementia at the same time, making diagnosis and predicting the course of the dementia symptoms more challenging. There are subtle features that differentiate the different types of dementia that your doctor can use to help better understand the type a patient has. For example, one of the discriminating features of Alzheimer's versus vascular dementia is that people with vascular dementia preserve the ability to name objects and the MRI often shows small vessel ischemia. Patients with Lewy body dementia are more likely to have visual hallucinations, muscle rigidity, and to act out their dreams. Parkinson's precedes Parkinson's dementia by about ten years. Creutzfeldt-Jakob is rapidly progressive to death within one year. Normal pressure hydrocephalus is unique in that it is preceded by urinary incontinence and trouble walking before the cognitive challenges. Lastly, Wernicke-Korsakoff syndrome is associated with heavy alcohol use and poor balance, and patients with this syndrome readily make up false stories with fairly quick speech (rapid verbal fluency).

To definitively know what type of dementia a person has, a brain biopsy is necessary. Since the brain biopsy does not change how the disease is treated and is very risky, it is recommended that the biopsy be conducted after death to provide grieving family members with closure and information about their family history.

You can't change your age, and you can't change your genes . . . at least not yet. But here is what you can do to maintain cognitive function.

What You Can Do for Yourself

- You guessed it! Eat a healthy diet and exercise daily.
- Avoid tobacco, alcohol, marijuana, and illicit drugs.
- People with MCI and dementia are particularly sensitive to medication and should avoid the following:
    - Benzodiazepines such as alprazolam (Xanax®), diazepam (Valium®), and lorazepam (Ativan®)
    - Anticholinergic medications—oxybutynin (Ditropan®), scopolamine (Dramamine®), Solifenacin (Vesicare®), and tolterodine (Detrol®)
    - Antihistamines—such as diphenhydramine (Benadryl®)
    - Opioids—such as oxycodone, hydrocodone, codeine, morphine, and dilaudid
- Work with your doctor to treat diabetes mellitus, high cholesterol (hyperlipidemia), high blood pressure (hypertension), and cardiovascular disease as they each affect blood flow to the brain.
- Obesity increases the risk of dementia by 50 percent, so work with your local gym and doctor to lose weight.
- Remain socially active.
- Seek treatment for depression, difficulty walking (gait impairments), and hearing loss as they lead to social isolation that increases the risk of dementia and mild cognitive impairment.
- Talk to your doctor about obstructive sleep apnea and any sleep disturbances to limit fatigue.
- It is unclear how much cognitive rehabilitation programs like Lumosity® work, but they aren't going to hurt, and they can be fun. Continue to stretch your brain by learning new things, reading, and doing puzzles. In fact, dancing is thought to be one of the best activities for your brain as you get exercise and have to learn and practice new steps! (Get ready to wow the grandkids with your hip-hop steps!)
- Occupational therapy (often covered by insurance) can help patients and caregivers with coping behaviors and strategies to compensate for deficits. This has been shown to have enduring benefits.

- Modify your environment by reducing the clutter and noise.
- Get a dry-erase board to outline the day's activities.
- To aid memory, write everything down . . . in one place! Perhaps a special notebook, one that also has a calendar.
- Stick to a routine and develop habits while you still have good cognitive function. A nighttime ritual is the most important.
- If needed, break down complex tasks into easier, smaller steps. For example, if you tell someone with dementia to brush their teeth, they may resist out of confusion. That is a very complex task. Try breaking the task down. Ask them first to pick up the toothpaste, then take the cap off the toothpaste, then pick up the toothbrush, then put toothpaste on the toothbrush, then put down the toothpaste, then turn on the water faucet, then put the toothbrush under the running water . . .
- Vitamin E (2,000 IU/day) has been studied with mixed results, showing possible benefit for dementia, but patients died at a younger age from other causes (higher all-cause mortality). It also doesn't appear to work with memantine mentioned below. Vitamin E may increase prostate cancer risks, so be sure to talk to your doctor before you embark on any treatment.
- Curcumin, which is in turmeric, has shown benefit in very small studies. There is definitely more for us to learn here.
- Consider music, pet, massage, and art therapy.
- Talk to family and friends and plan for the future. You may need a support group, legal advisers, and new members for your medical team.
- More research is needed before the effectiveness of estrogen replacement, selegiline, anti-inflammatory medication, ginkgo biloba, statins, super vitamin B, and omega-3 fatty acids can be determined.
- Safety can become a major issue, and concerns around driving, wandering, and living alone must be discussed. I often recommend having family members unplug the stove and disconnect the car battery, when cooking and driving are no longer safe, to allow patients to stay home safely longer.
- Oversight of financial management is highly recommended before elder financial abuse is discovered too late.

- Even if your cognitive function is normal, there is a good chance that you have a mate who is struggling. Support groups can be so helpful. Learn as much as you can about dementia from books like *The 36 Hour Day* and *Ahead of Dementia.* Caregiving is hard. Get therapy to support yourself and your own well-being. Talk to members of your spiritual community. Continue to spend time with family and friends. Ask for help. There are many helpful tips on how to assist your loved one and yourself.

What Your Doctor Can Do

- Provide advice and accountability on diet and exercise.
- Help you manage any diabetes, cardiovascular disease, high blood pressure (hypertension), and/or high cholesterol (hyperlipidemia).
- Help you treat your depression or make referrals for therapy and treatment.
- Refer you to an audiologist so that you can stay socially active.
- Refer you to physical therapy so that you can remain mobile and engaged in your world.
- Diagnose and treat sleep disorders.
- Make referrals to occupational therapy to teach adaptation skills.
- For mild to moderate dementia, your doctor may recommend cholinesterase inhibitors like donepezil (Aricept®), rivastigmine (Exelon®), and galantamine (Razadyne®) that provide modest effects, slowing decline on cognitive tests and some global impression by caregivers. The thought is that they prevent two months per year of decline compared to a typical patient with Alzheimer's who is not treated. I do prescribe these medications for my patients. I try to start them early in the disease process. If patients develop side effects and I have to stop them, I don't feel like much has been lost.
- When a patient reaches the stage of moderate dementia, memantine (Namenda®) is often added. It can also be used

without a cholinesterase inhibitor if a patient had to stop using them.
- Your doctor may prescribe other medications to treat symptoms that arise from dementia like depression, sleep disturbances, hallucinations, or agitation.

You might be wondering why I didn't mention the medication aducanumab. It was just announced in public media at the time this book was being finalized. As of right now, there is much controversy over this new medication that aims to slow the declines associated with Alzheimer's disease. Its release created much excitement because it is the first medication to be released for Alzheimer's in over seventeen years, the results from the scientific studies were underwhelming, and the price tag was enough to potentially bankrupt Medicare at $56,000 per person per year. Needless to say, this story has only begun to be written.

Still with Gifts to Give

One of my favorite patients to visit is 102 years old. She played competitive tennis until she was ninety-four. Now she sings and dances. I love to go visit her. We always start by singing together—first "Take Me Out to the Ball Game" and then circle around to "Que Sera, Sera," run through a series of old famous musical hits, and end with "Seventy-Six Trombones" from *The Music Man*. She doesn't really *need* her walker; it is more of a dance partner when I or others are not available. She has Alzheimer's dementia, and it is severe. She lives in an assisted living community with a twenty-four-hour caregiver who takes her down for community meals and events every day. She radiates joy, and it is contagious. Even the grumpiest of old men at the facility smile as she literally waltzes by their table. Her eighty-year-old daughter and I often talk about how she enlivens everyone's spirit. She is such an asset to her community, dementia and all.

I have only known her since her dementia was so severe that she no longer knew what she had lost. But I have known many others watch themselves go through the process of realization, some getting lost in grief and bitterness. I have seen others choose the path that they wanted for themselves. Enjoying their puzzles and games, whether they help or not. Continuing to socialize and learning to laugh at themselves. Using their clothes to project how they wanted to be seen. Setting physical challenges for themselves each week at the gym, that people twenty years their junior admired. They demonstrated a willingness to adopt new techniques to help their memory, not fighting change but asking for help when needed. They were determined to choose a path of least resistance and let go a little for their own greater happiness. They are becoming my 102-year-old.

I have plenty of patients with all of the risk factors for dementia, but knowing they were getting older and had a parent with Alzheimer's or other forms of dementia, they worked to keep their bad (LDL) cholesterol down low, they exercised regularly, ate whole, unprocessed foods (food without labels!), continued to take adult education classes to stimulate their brains, watched their weight, and avoided anything that could negatively affect their cognition. Hundreds of these patients escaped getting dementia. Were they just lucky? I'd like to think they earned it. This is not to say that it is 100 percent preventable, but sometimes, it certainly is or can at least be delayed.

CHAPTER TWENTY
RETIREMENT: ARE YOU REALLY READY?

Freedom

No, I'm not talking about whether or not you have saved enough money to stop working. I'm a physician, and despite years of education, I have never taken a business course or finance class, so let's leave that topic to the professional financial planners. A doctor's job is to ensure that you are mentally ready to retire. Have you prepared for what you are going to do after retirement? A five- to twenty-year vacation from work will quickly take its toll on your mental and physical health if you don't have a plan before you leave your career.

My father-in-law worked for the local city's wastewater treatment plant for decades and retired at seventy-five. Fortunately, he had been a runner, and he transitioned to hiking, which maintains his physical fitness. As a quiet, introverted, single man, we worried about how he would manage socially, leaving his friends of decades, and we encouraged him to make a retirement plan.

The plan can certainly start with six months of celebration, naps, impromptu visits with friends, random adventures, and no structured activities. You will deserve time to recover from years of a rigid, hectic, high-pressured and structured working life, but that period of celebration must have an end date. At some point, after the initial thrill of retirement has just begun to fade, consider doing the following:

What You Can Do for Yourself

- Establish a weekly exercise regime that includes aerobic exercise (e.g., walking, biking, etc.), balance and stretching exercises, and weightlifting (even if it is two to three pounds!).
- Follow your passions (e.g., consider volunteering, taking classes for seniors, etc.).
- Develop your favorite hobby (e.g., practice the piano, continue painting, etc.).
- Plan regular social activities with friends and family. This may be a time to build your friend network if you have lost your daily work friends.
- Create a bucket list of things you want to do or accomplish in your lifetime.
- Replace old work routines with new daily routines (e.g., go to sleep and wake up at the same time every day, exercise daily, etc.).
- Share your retirement plans with your spouse, friends, and family.

Get Creative

For some, you may want to get creative with these activities. Joni volunteers at a pet shelter and frequently fosters dogs. She currently is helping a very large but too skinny German shepherd recover from a heartworm infection. The German shepherd is very well socialized and is able to go for long walks, which Joni does with her retired neighbors during the week and her working friends on the weekends. She gets to volunteer helping dogs, which provides structure to her week and is her passion, and she socializes with others while getting exercise. Oh, and the dog wakes her up at 7 am every day!

Jack is a Holocaust survivor who readily shares his personal story and message of respect for all human beings. Currently in his nineties, he is a well-known speaker who continues to speak to large audiences. Sharing his message for the benefit of others is his passion; it keeps him connected to the greater community and provides him with a routine that so many others can benefit from.

Stages of Retirement

It is also helpful to know and anticipate the stages of retirement.

Stage 1: Pre-Retirement

Before retirement, take time to imagine what you are going to do with your new life. How are you going to spend your time? Some people take five to ten years to plan their retirement. They may plan a move to a new location or save money for a special trip. While you are planning your finances, don't forget to plan for fun activities and how you will find purpose in these years of your life.

Stage 2: Honeymoon Phase

This period starts the day you retire and can last six months to two years. People feel liberated, excited, relieved, and free of stress and the burdens of work. Many people spend this time reconnecting with people, participating in hobbies, traveling, and starting small side businesses.

Stage 3: Disenchantment

After the honeymoon comes a period of disenchantment and disillusionment. People often feel boredom, loneliness, and lose their sense of purpose. If it is not anticipated and planned for, it can easily turn into a period of depression.

Stage 4: Recovering

At this point, one must research for purpose, goals, and create their new identity that will allow them to truly transition from their work-self to their retired-self. This is the stage that people find who they will be for the rest of their life.

Stage 5: Stability

Retirees at this stage are content and hopeful. They have found a fun and rewarding retirement lifestyle for themselves that makes them feel fulfilled. It is focused on maintaining their health, connecting with others, participating in purposeful activities, and having an established routine.

As I sit here, my spouse is trying to learn how to crochet with yarn in one hand, a crocheting needle in the other, and a series of YouTube videos. Perhaps, she is in Stage 1: preparing for retirement. Seniors who engage in these seven activities listed above are happier and are less likely to suffer from anxiety and depression than those who don't have a routine or a plan. They are physically healthier and able to live independently for longer. They move through the stages of retirement with more ease. Hopefully, that's all the motivation you need to reconsider your retirement plan! Before I retire from practicing medicine to my dream retirement world of writing, I just hope that I'll have a new crocheted hat!

CHAPTER TWENTY-ONE
GRIEF AND LOSS: HOW MUCH MORE CAN I LOSE?

Purpose in Life

I learned something new about one of my patients this week, and it made me so sad. I have known this eighty-year-old husband and wife couple for several years. Despite a few aches and pains from arthritis, a recent hip replacement for her, and an irregular heartbeat (atrial fibrillation) in him, I am always impressed by how active they are. Specifically, he walks six miles a day, takes singing lessons, and plays the clarinet. He is a father and grandfather who has a close relationship with his family. He is on several organizational boards in the city and is very politically active.

At his most recent visit, his wife joined him for his annual physical. As spouses often do, she gave away one of his deepest secrets. (This time, it wasn't that he eats too much cake and ice cream.) He feels that ever since he retired he has no purpose in his life. When I heard that, my heart sank.

I always enjoy seeing him. He makes me smile. I love hearing his nostalgic accent and sharing stories. He is a fellow New Yorker here in Denver, and I feel like he is the only one around who roots for the same sports teams as me. I feel like we have a deep, unspoken connection on some level. He is a wonderful man, and I am sure that he connects with others as well. How can he not see that he contributes to my world? And to others, I'm sure! His calming, even presence helps ground his highly energetic wife. The way they talk about their children and grandchildren, it is clear that they have a relationship that he is very much an integral part of. He brings music to his audiences, knowledge, experience, and connections to his organizational boards, and played a role in the most recent election, in which the candidates he supported got elected. Yet, he no longer feels like he is contributing. He continues to feel like he had lost everything when he retired.

Now, let me tell you about a different man that I saw today for a follow-up visit. This gentleman, whom I will call Jay, is ninety years old. Advanced age and declining health have left him blind in both eyes and with little use of his left hand, which he calls his claw. Fortunately, he is right-handed, and his right arm and hand are still functional. He has a huge, severe (Stage 4) pressure wound (decubitus ulcer) on his buttocks. His legs are too weak to walk or stand for now. He is bedridden. I no longer visit him at home for his care, but instead, I see him at the long-term acute care hospital where he resides while his wound heals.

During our last conversation, he talked about how difficult the transition from a highly independent businessman to his current state of total dependence has become. He recounted that on his many business trips, he was so independent that, unlike many husbands of his generation, he always packed his luggage even though he knew his wife of decades "knew [him] well enough to do a perfect job packing." Then, he repeated twice, "I am totally dependent. I am *totally* dependent." The comment was more reflective than sorrowful.

After a very short pause, he said with a lift in his voice and a smile on his face, "It is remarkable how much I can do by just feeling with my right hand. I don't think people realize just how important the sense of touch is."

Through our conversation, he proceeded to tell me about the relationships he had developed with his caregivers. The one that seemed most meaningful was with a Black male nurse. He recalled how he insisted that the nurse call him by his first name. The nurse commented that twenty years ago, calling a white man by their first name was not acceptable, and it was a difficult habit to break. From there, they were able to engage in a deep and meaningful conversation about race and race relations. Jay is quick to inspire and encourage profound, thoughtful, and productive dialogue on topics related to social justice, politics, history, and current events. He has a long road ahead of him, with multiple upcoming surgeries. He could easily throw in the towel, but he feels like he has more to contribute to the world, and he is not yet ready to concede. Selfishly, I want to hear more of what he has to say!

Patient Wisdom

Each and every individual responds to loss differently, and each loss is unique. But what is inevitable is that, over time, the losses accumulate. One of my patients provided what I thought was a most valuable analogy to loss. She had lost her husband years ago and was happily remarried for well over a decade. She said, "They tell you that after you lose a spouse, the pain of the loss gets smaller over time. But that is not true. I think of losing my spouse like a hole in a tapestry. That hole never goes away, and it never gets smaller. Instead, over my lifetime, I continue to sew a bigger tapestry so that the hole is proportionally a smaller piece of my life."

Another patient who lost her husband said, "I was married to a most wonderful, curious, creative man. He loved life and loved exploration and discovery. When he died, it was crushing, but I knew that I wanted to honor him, and the only way to do that was to celebrate life as he did. I miss him every day. There is a void that will never be filled. And that's okay. I am so grateful for the life we had together and all the lovely memories. I am open to life and its ever-changingness. Who knows what the future holds, and isn't that exciting?"

This same patient quoted her mom, who would say, "Life by the yard is hard. Life by the inch is a cinch." When life is difficult, take it one day at a time, or just one step at a time.

Loneliness

Loss often leads to loneliness. Perhaps it is the loss of relatives, friends, and neighbors. Even if an elderly person has miraculously not lost a single soul to death, as mentioned above, there is functional loss that leads to loneliness. Does loss of hearing make it harder to connect with others? Have you stopped meeting with friends and family because you find the trips too fatiguing or because it is too hard to navigate out of your home? Loneliness can be experienced whether you are surrounded by people or are alone. In total, 11 percent of all people report being lonely, but 43 percent of people over the age of sixty acknowledge loneliness.

Loneliness not only doesn't feel good, but it negatively affects your health. It increases your fight-or-flight hormones (adrenaline and norepinephrine), which stresses the body, leads to fatigue, causes anxiety or just a jittery unsettled feeling, and results in insomnia. It increases pain perception in the brain, decreases the immune system's ability to fight infection, and decreases sleep quality. Loneliness is a risk factor for many diseases such as coronary artery disease, diabetes mellitus, osteoarthritis, Alzheimer's dementia, and more.

Loneliness, sadness, or grief from loss is normal and can be quite severe in the short term. These reactions are normal responses to life events such as bereavement, adjustments to changes in social status with retirement and loss of income, transitioning from independent living to assisted living or residential care, and loss of physical, social, or cognitive function. The problem occurs when these feelings last long, one fails to recover to a new semblance of life, and/or their loneliness, sadness, or grief progresses to a depressive disorder. Some people have worsening depression as they age, while others experience it for the first time. Those at highest risk for depression are females, those who are socially isolated, widowed, or living alone, and/or have medical problems, uncontrolled pain, insomnia, functional impairment, and/or cognitive impairment. Many older people have most of these risk factors.

What You Can Do for Yourself

What should you do if you are experiencing loss, loneliness, grief, depression, or anxiety? There are three levels of approach, and they all intersect: self-help techniques, therapy, and medication (see Figure 21.1). Self-help is a great place to start for loneliness. If you notice that your symptoms are affecting your ability to function and do the things you want to do or usually do in a day, then be sure to read the tips in Chapter 22. Loneliness and grief can evolve into depression and anxiety.

Self-Help Tips

This entire book has included self-help tips. This section is no different. Bookstores are filled with books on how to guide personal improvement, because education is power, and people want to empower themselves to

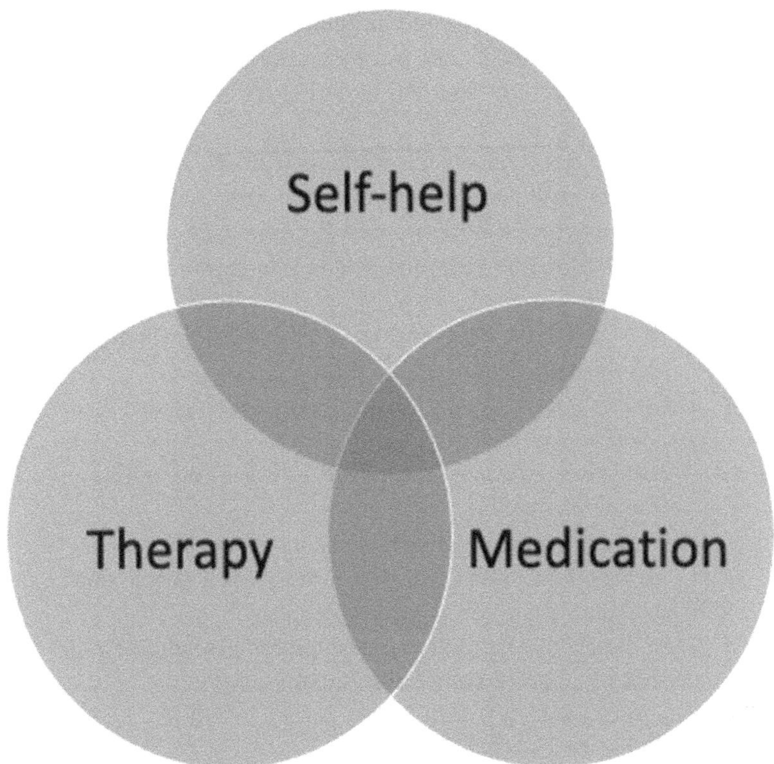

Figure 21.1. A Venn diagram demonstrating the treatment options for loss, loneliness, grief, depression and anxiety.

improve their situation. Here are some suggestions in regard to loss, loneliness, and the resulting depression and anxiety that you can employ to feel better.

What You Can Do for Yourself

- Always be kind to yourself.
- Limit alcohol and caffeine.
- Eat well-balanced meals.
- Get enough sleep.
- Exercise daily and practice de-stressing–yoga, deep breathing, meditation, etc.

- Exercise generates hope, happiness, a sense of purpose, greater life satisfaction, and connection with others.
- Build structure into your day or week, and try to stick to a routine.
- When you feel good about something, share it.
  - Create small moments of connection with others.
- Reach out to people in close proximity, or strengthen weak ties to others, focus on others, and tend to your network of friends and contacts.
  - If you haven't been talking, it takes time to find your words. Be patient with yourself.
- Do more things with people, and choose the things that make you feel connected.
  - Do lunch, talk on Zoom, Skype, or FaceTime, and/or go for a walk together.
  - If you don't enjoy sitting and talking, invite others to participate in activities with you instead. Most people don't talk during a movie, a concert, or a play!
- Take the actions you need to feel better, being mindful of your personality and values when choosing these actions.
- Find your passion(s).
  - What do you value?
  - What does your social world look like to you, and how do you experience it?
  - Do you have supportive relationships with family and friends?
  - Are there local formal or informal social groups to which you belong or could join?
  - Are there factors that prevent social connection, such as a lack of transport?
  - Have you experienced a recent significant change in your life (e.g., bereavement, a move, retiring, ill health, etc.)?
  - What are your hopes and dreams for the future?
  - What have you always wanted to do?
  - How do you get there?

- Underactivity leads to internal chatter that is often self-destructive, while overactivity is often a sign of avoidance of internal emotions; find the balance.

What Your Doctor Can Do

- See if you would benefit from treatment with a therapist or medications.
- Assess the level of your suffering and see if you have depression or anxiety.

Truly Alone

This week, I met another older woman whose only family member was a nephew 1,000 miles away, whom I have not been able to reach by phone. I asked her if she had any friends, and she said that she talked to her insurance agent and postman . . . it is so important to continue to make connections and to stay involved with your community at whatever level is comfortable for you as you age or to reach out to groups that provide companionship. There are so many lonely elders that could be connected to each other.

Now, remember the story of the tapestry from earlier in the chapter. After each loss, we need to work to make our tapestry bigger. For my family, we fill our home with dogs and cats. We fill our lives with family and friends. We spend our time helping others, delivering fresh home-baked pies, and writing. That is the way we connect to our community. We spend time hiking in the mountains and stretching our bodies to stay in tune with nature and what our bodies still can do. It all helps make the losses a relatively smaller portion of our growing lives. What are you doing to make your tapestry bigger?

CHAPTER TWENTY-TWO

DEPRESSION AND ANXIETY: TWO SIDES OF THE SAME COIN

I remember being taught in residency that depression and anxiety are two sides of the same coin. While an oversimplification, depression results from worrying about the past, and anxiety results from worrying about the future. Genetic research and enhanced brain imaging such as functional MRI are starting to demonstrate the link between these two disorders. This may explain why many people suffer from both.

Increasingly, I am seeing older patients come to my office expressing concerns over their personal depression and anxiety or seeing these symptoms in their loved ones. This brings me great relief. For so many years, the stigma around mental health diseases and disorders prevented patients from seeking help, and instead, they suffered needlessly. Now, I don't want to give the misperception that these diseases are easily and quickly treated, but there are treatments that make the symptoms more tolerable and the course of illness shorter, thereby decreasing suffering.

Honestly, you will notice that this chapter is very similar to the loneliness chapter because the way I look at grief and loneliness is very similar. Many life events lead to mental health challenges, whether or not they rise to the level of a diagnosable illness. I do know that loss at any age can exacerbate depression and anxiety, and that as one ages, losses start to really accumulate.

Meera presented to me almost paralyzed with depression. She had been living in Washington, DC, until her husband died eighteen months ago. She decided to move to Denver to be closer to her only child and grandchildren, but then the COVID-19 lockdowns left her confined to her new tiny apartment in an unfamiliar city where she had only her daughter and no friends or siblings. Then her son-in-law caught COVID-19 at work and lost his hearing, leaving him disabled. The daughter, overwhelmed by her new role as a caretaker of her husband and children, was no longer available to emotionally support her mother, Meera, who had a relapse of her major depression.

Gino is a dedicated and loving husband of fifty-four years to his wife, Josie. Josie, however, is progressing from moderate to severe Alzheimer's, and the tears fill his eyes and anxiety fills his mind when he thinks about leaving the house, even for a moment. "What if she wakes up and asks for me and I'm not there?" His anxiety is preventing him from taking care of himself, even though their children have come to the house to watch mom and to take him for lunch or to the grocery store. His anxiety keeps him trapped in his home. My suggestion that the daughter could just respond to mom's concerns by saying, "Dad is at the store and will be right back," seems incomprehensible or perhaps reprehensible.

Depression and Anxiety

There are many types of depressive disorders, such as major depressive disorder, seasonal affective disorder, adjustment disorder, and dysthymia. Symptoms include sadness, having little interest in doing things that you previously enjoyed, and social regression. Other symptoms seen in younger individuals with depression may be less diagnostic in the elderly, such as sleeping too much or too little all of a sudden, changes to your appetite, moving slowly, trouble concentrating, and thoughts of death. Some older people want to hurt themselves or commit suicide, and that warrants urgent medical intervention. Men with depression are more likely to abuse substances like alcohol in attempts to self-treat their symptoms, making their symptoms harder to recognize. They tend to be more irritable, angry, and tired. Women, on the other hand, are more likely to ruminate, feel sad, worthless, or guilty, and become depressed from increasing burdens of stress. Women also tend to experience accompanying anxiety with their depression.

Symptoms of anxiety include feeling nervous or anxious, not being able to stop worrying, trouble relaxing, feeling restless, becoming easily annoyed or irritable, and/or feeling like something awful might happen. Men have as much anxiety as women, but like depression, they often try to self-medicate, making it harder to recognize. Men with anxiety are more likely to report strained relationships with friends and family and are more likely to fear social consequences of their anxiety. Women tend to have a greater burden of illness when they have anxiety and are more likely to have associated headaches, fatigue, muscle tension, and heart, lung, and gastrointestinal symptoms.

Mental Health and Physical Health

As an aside, I want to talk about how mental health issues are different from physical health issues. Well, last time I checked, our brains were connected to our bodies. In fact, all of the common chemicals that cause depression, anxiety, grief, loneliness—serotonin, dopamine, norepinephrine—have receptors not just in the brain but throughout our bodies. This helps explain, for example, why anxiety can cause palpitations and depression can cause weakness, fatigue, and changes in bowel habits, among other symptoms. The only difference between mental health issues and physical health issues is how they have been unfortunately divided in our culture. There is no difference. My biggest fear is that if I say, "I think your chest discomfort is from your anxiety," you will hear, "My doctor thinks that it is all in my head." I want you to know that other doctors and I see it as a legitimate explanation for your symptoms.

See Table 22.1, which illustrates where all of the "brain" chemicals also work outside your brain. Changes to any of these chemicals can cause symptoms in those respective organs throughout your body.

What You Can Do for Yourself

What should you do if you are experiencing depression or anxiety? There are three levels of approach, and they all intersect: self-help techniques, therapy, and medication (see Figure 21.1 from the last chapter).

Table 22.1. Locations where different "brain" chemicals also affect how organs function.

Serotonin	*Norepinephrine*	*Dopamine*
Brain	Brain	Brain
Arteries	Lymph nodes	Lymph nodes
Muscles	Heart	Arteries
Stomach	Arteries	Spleen
Intestines	Muscles	Stomach
Platelets	Stomach	Pancreas
Nerves	Liver	Intestines
	Pancreas	Kidneys
	Spleen	
	Intestines	
	Fat	

Self-Help Tips

This entire book has included self-help tips. This section is no different as for loneliness but keep reading! Bookstores are filled with books on how to guide personal improvement, because education is power, and people want to empower themselves to improve their situation. Here are some suggestions in regard to loss, loneliness, and resulting depression and anxiety that you can employ to feel better.

What You Can Do for Yourself

- Always be kind to yourself.
- Limit alcohol and caffeine.
- Eat well-balanced meals.
- Get enough sleep . . . but not too much.
- Exercise daily and practice de-stressing–yoga, deep-breathing, meditation, etc.
    - Exercise generates hope, happiness, a sense of purpose, greater life satisfaction, and connection with others.
- Build structure into your day or week and try to stick to a routine.

- Reach out to people in close proximity or strengthen weak ties to others, focus on others, and tend to your network of friends and contacts.
- Take the actions you need to feel better, being mindful of your personality and values when choosing these actions.
- Underactivity leads to internal chatter that is often self-destructive, while overactivity is often a sign of avoidance of internal emotions; find the balance.

Therapy

Therapy is essential for most people with depression, always for anxiety, and has been shown to be very effective. It is underutilized in late-life depression and anxiety, especially given its tremendous benefit. I do want to point out though that it may be less effective in people who have severe dementia, at which point I would recommend that you spend the money on therapy for their caregivers! There are many different types of therapy. If you have a preference, go with that type; otherwise, start with cognitive behavioral therapy (CBT) or psychodynamic psychotherapy.

What Will a Therapist Do?

- Therapy will help you feel your feelings so you can manage them, make you aware of patterns that you didn't see before, help you to be more self-accepting, and feel less alone.
- It is a slow process (months to years), and it is expensive but will likely be the best money you have ever spent.
- Seeing a therapist is not a sign of weakness. You do not have to be crazy to see a therapist or to benefit from what they have to offer. If you struggle with the idea of seeing a therapist, think of them as a life coach. Most high-level executive positions in business come with a business or executive coach; athletes work with sports psychologists, why not have one for the hardest job, managing life?

CHAPTER TWENTY-TWO

Medications

Medications have also been found to be effective and are recommended for moderate to severe symptoms. Medications can take four to six weeks to work if you have never taken them before. For most people, medications work much, much, much better when people are also in therapy. Yes, these medications have side effects . . . but they get better with time and are often well worth the wait. I have found that the minor passing side effects pale in comparison to the struggle of depression and anxiety. Most people do not need to be on these medications for the rest of their lives. I tend to prescribe them for about eighteen to twenty-four months after an episode of depression and then reassess the need to continue.

What Your Doctor Can Do

- Your doctor can assess the severity of your symptoms and let you know if it is time for medication.
- Your doctor can recommend a therapist to work with. If you don't feel like it is a good fit between you and the therapist, don't give up. Try someone else.
- Most antidepressant and antianxiety medications work on serotonin and norepinephrine. The simple way to think about them is that serotonin is the "feel good" hormone, which is why SSRI medications like fluoxetine (Prozac®), escitalopram (Lexapro®), citalopram (Celexa®), and sertraline (Zoloft®) help with depression. I don't use paroxetine (Paxil®) as much in the elderly due to the side effects.
- The simple way to think about norepinephrine is that it is the "energy and alertness" hormone. People who need to feel good and need a boost of energy benefit from the SNRI category of antidepressants, such as venlafaxine (Effexor®), desvenlafaxine (Pristiq®), and duloxetine (Cymbalta®).
- There are also several other antidepressants that are effective that don't fit neatly into these two categories, which is why a discussion with your doctor is best to help choose which medication would be best for you. I also like using mirtazapine (Remeron®) for older patients because it also helps with

appetite and insomnia. Bupropion (Wellbutrin®) is another medication that I have had a lot of success using with my patients, especially those who have daytime fatigue and lethargy. Even then, it is not always clear which type will work best for you, so you might have to try more than one. Vilazodone (Viibryd®) and vortioxetine (Trintellix®) have some of the least sexual side effects if that is an unwelcome side effect of other medications. Of note, medications that have helped family members are more likely to help you too. If you know what worked for your sibling's depression, it is most likely going to work for you as well.

- Your doctor can work with you to decide which medication would be best for you.
- A word of caution: don't just stop antidepressant and antianxiety medications when you are feeling better, unless instructed to do so! Most of these medications need to be tapered off over weeks. If you feel that you are ready to stop a medication or need to do so because of a side effect, your doctor can help.

Suicidal Thoughts

Some elderly people do struggle with thoughts of suicide, and they can be quite successful in their attempts to end their lives. Elderly patients with suicidal thoughts require immediate medical referral (call their doctor immediately). People who are experiencing hallucinations and/or seeing, hearing, smelling, or feeling people or things that others don't or are not there need to seek medical attention to determine the cause. Hallucinations can be caused by depression and other psychiatric conditions but also by strokes and seizures as well. These conditions can be treated.

Denial

Denial around mental illness is rampant. I had a physician patient, whom I have a lot of respect for as a colleague and human being, present to my office with debilitating fatigue after stopping Zoloft®. He had started the medication two years prior to help with the grief and sadness that followed his wife's prolonged death from cancer. He insisted that his fatigue was coming from deep inside and must have a medical cause. After an extensive workup, no cause was found. After months, he was finally agreeable to restarting Zoloft®, at which point his fatigue disappeared. Was he willing to acknowledge that he had fatigue from depression, now gone once he was back on Zoloft®? No. His response was, "Well, I'm glad the fatigue is gone, but I guess we will never know what caused it."

When patients are going through such a really tough time and there are resources to help, be it therapy or medicine, it pains me to see them suffer as opposed to taking advantage of effective treatment. According to the Centers for Disease Control, depression and anxiety in the elderly are as high as 15 to 20 percent. Many, many patients seek mental health support. But because no one talks about it, everyone thinks that they are the only ones who are struggling and are in need of external assistance. Hopefully, I just corrected that myth, so now you won't be shy about talking to your doctor.

CHAPTER TWENTY-THREE
RESILIENCY: BE A RUBBER BALL

Bounce

My mother would often reminisce about a game she played with her great-grandfather when she was a small child. When she went to her great-grandfather's home, he would have a rubber ball set aside and a single shiny penny. To play the game, he would sit in a lawn chair on the cement patio, and she would stand about eight feet away. Between them, on the ground would rest the shiny penny. They would then bounce the rubber handball back and forth to each other, trying to hit the penny, scoring one point each time the penny moved! It was a simple game for a grandparent to play with their grandchild, and it left wonderful, happy, lasting memories. It was also a game that I played with my grandmother and mother.

What made the rubber ball so much fun in this game was that it bounced. Despite being thrown to the ground, being disfigured with each impact, it always rebounded. It demonstrated great resilience, as did my competitive relatives who sometimes lost the game. It was a great way for my mother to develop a relationship with her great-grandparents who only spoke a language she didn't understand: Italian. It was also a great way for him to play with his great-grandchildren even though he could no longer run around like he used to.

When I joined my partner, David Mellman, MD, in practice, he was already sending quarterly newsletters to his patients. With the help of his wife, Pippa, we added a monthly educational series where we would have a group of patients to their home for afternoon tea to discuss a medical topic. Pippa was born in England, and though she moved to the United States as a child, the idea of us serving afternoon English tea with cucumber sandwiches, berries, and scones piqued the interest of our patients.

Our first topics included aging, women's health, men's health, and pre-diabetes. I'm not sure what the patients enjoyed most, the topic information, getting a chance to interact with their doctor outside of the office, gathering with community members that they hadn't seen in years, making new friends, or the tasty tea and scones.

Months later, when COVID-19 struck our community, people were being asked to physically distance themselves. At the same time, the country was experiencing political and social unrest, great social divides, and a failing economy, plus individual personal tragedies. Everything about the world seemed unpredictable and uncertain. We were concerned about the well-being of our patient community. We moved the talks to a less intimate setting online but appreciated the safety from COVID-19 that Zoom provided. As I mentioned earlier, I started writing weekly newsletters that included information on various health topics and included responses to any questions that patients had submitted the week prior via email. I didn't know what else to do, and I thought at least the newsletters might help our patients to feel connected during a time of physical isolation.

Reflecting on Resilience

During this period, I would have entire days where every patient appointment was directly related to the stress of COVID-19 and related lifestyle changes. Patients presented with anxiety, fear, depression, loneliness, helplessness, fatigue, lack of motivation, marital strain, worry over their children and grandchildren, feeling overwhelmed, financial stress, and despair from job loss. Other patients came in for their usual check-ups and seemed to be taking all of the turmoil and change in stride.

It made me reflect on what resilience is and what makes some people more resilient. I started by reading a series of articles in the *New York Times* about resilience and reflected on what I had learned approximately twenty years ago about surviving residency training. Resilience is the ability to recover from difficult experiences, setbacks, and tragedies and to be able to move forward, learn, adapt, and grow from one's challenges. The first patient that I lost unexpectedly as a resident was 102 years old. He came into the hospital with congestive heart failure. I was giving him medicine to take the extra fluid off of his heart. Each day, he was getting better. His labs were improving, and he felt great, and then unexpectedly, he died. The heart monitor he was on did not reveal any cause of death, and his family declined an autopsy. A loss of life is always difficult, and I was able to move forward and continue to take care of other patients that day, but I really wanted to know why he died. I called his primary care doctor, who was one of the smartest and most experienced doctors I knew because I wanted to understand for the benefit of subsequent patients. I wanted to grow as a person from every patient interaction. The great doctor said to me, "Sometimes, people's bodies just wear out, and they die. Don't think so hard. He was 102." That in and of itself was a lesson that I had never read in a medical school textbook. Every loss, every challenge, and every mistake has made me a better doctor, as I strive to learn and grow from each human interaction.

How to Reach Ninety-Two

Then I remembered a conversation I had with yet another one of my physically and mentally healthy patients in their nineties. Nancy is a ninety-two-year-old woman, and I asked her that cliché question, "How does one get to be ninety-two years old?" She responded, "I work out three times a day. I do forty-five minutes of stretching in the morning, forty-five minutes of weights in the afternoon, and forty-five minutes of treadmill in the evening. Don't you wish you were retired too?" Her inspirational story is where I find my resilience. I am inspired by my patients every day. It is because of them that I exercise even when I don't want to.

I currently have several Holocaust survivors in my practice that have a will to live like no other. Throughout my career, I have watched tens of thousands of patients, some more resilient than others, and I couldn't help but wonder if it wasn't in part genetic. Well, as it turns out, genetics plays a very, very small part in one's degree of resilience. While genetics influence temperament, personality, and diseases like depression, anxiety, and PTSD, there doesn't seem to be a genetic link to resiliency. This may be because resiliency is a trait, and almost any trait can be either positive or negative, depending on the situation.

Say, for example, you are hiking in the forest when you spot a wild animal. If you are genetically inclined to be impulsive or anxious or quick to startle and take off running, this might be an advantage if you encounter a squirrel protecting its nest but not if you encounter a bear protecting its cubs.

Resilience Can Be Learned

As it turns out, resilience is taught and can be learned! It is a set of skills that are learned from exposure to a series of very challenging but manageable experiences of increasing difficulty. As a resident on a busy call night in the hospital, I learned that if I could cope with all that was happening, then by the next day, I would be stronger and able to handle more. The actual story went like this: I was a second-year medical resident, and it was my first night alone in the hospital without any senior physicians. I did have a brand-new intern who had just graduated from medical school, but I knew all of the decisions, procedures, and life-saving code blues were my responsibility and that I had a team to lead. The way our hospital worked, I had already been working for ten hours when all of the other doctors left for the day. Within fifteen minutes, I was called with fourteen patients that needed to be admitted from the emergency department to the hospital. They each needed to be seen, evaluated, have their medications ordered, test and labs ordered, diets chosen, IV drips requested, consults called, and therapy requests placed. For two minutes, I was paralyzed and overwhelmed with the volume of work and the fear that I could still get called with thirty more patients in the remaining hours of the night. After a deep breath to calm myself, I realized that I could only see them one at a time, and I asked the emergency room doctors and nurses to help me see the sickest people first. My intern and I survived that very busy night, and so did all of our patients! After that night, there wasn't anything that I couldn't handle. Each year of residency led to incrementally more responsibility and the development of more resilience. By the time I was done, I was ready for the mass casualties that I would encounter every few years in my career. And by 2020, I was ready for COVID-19.

People with more resilience often have a growth mindset rather than a fixed mindset. People with a fixed mindset see mistakes and challenges as signs of their own incompetence and failures, and they give up. Those with a growth mindset see each setback as a way to learn and as an opportunity for growth. Of course, we all have characteristics of both, but we tend to lean more towards one mindset than the other. If you bake a cake and it turns out poorly, do you figure out your error and try again, or do you give up and buy a cake instead?

People that are lucky enough to have quality, close personal relationships and parents that they could form early healthy attachments to find it easier to develop resilience. Attachment to others, especially at an early age, is crucial. If you are not sure if you had healthy relationships as a child or currently, ask yourself these questions: How loved did you feel as a child? How loved do you feel now? You would be surprised to learn how many adults have no close personal relationships.

Traumas and a person's age at the time of the traumas impact one's perception, interpretations, and expectations. This also has a great impact on how resilience is fostered, developed, and sustained. For example, if you lost your home in a hurricane but your family remained tightly supportive and you were able to move into secure housing and, eventually, a new home, you will experience resiliency differently than the person who loses their home and ends up homeless with their family. The impact on resilience is also very different for the trauma victim who is sexually abused as a child by a family member, loses their ability to rely on others, and is left to develop their own adaptive system of self-reliance. Some are more successful at becoming resilient than others, and that largely depends on other features of their surrounding environment.

Coping Mechanisms

When we are faced with challenges so great that we become overwhelmed, we must resort to coping mechanisms. I use the word "we" because it happens to all of us, all of the time. Some coping strategies are positive and adaptive, and some are maladaptive. We all use strategies from each list, with the intention of using less maladaptive strategies. I will admit that I indulged in a ridiculously large slice of apple pie (à la mode) this evening for all of the wrong reasons . . .

- Adaptive
    - Confronting problems directly
    - Making reasonable, realistic appraisals of problems
    - Recognizing and changing unhealthy emotional reactions
    - Mindfulness
    - Trying to prevent adverse effects on the body
    - Planning and following one's moral compass
    - Cognitive and emotional flexibility
    - Self-compassion
    - Optimism (positive reframing) and humor
    - Seeking care and reaching out for help in a healthy way
    - Social connectedness, with a degree of selflessness
- Maladaptive
    - Escaping problems, denial, avoidance
    - Distress
    - Anxiety
    - Blaming, venting
    - Risk-taking behaviors
    - Lying
    - Fear
    - Ruminating and perseverating
    - Dwelling on the negative
    - Physical symptoms

It turns out that these coping mechanisms become very deeply ingrained behavior patterns that are hard to change. But, it is not impossible! How mindful can you be of your actions and emotions to identify your own maladaptive behaviors? Can you consciously choose to replace them with an adaptive behavior instead? Most people need a life coach or a therapist to help make these changes.

What does this have to do with aging? Everything. Successful aging requires an incredible amount of resiliency because aging is full of change, challenges, setbacks, and obstacles. And there are benefits to consciously deciding how you are going to face these changes, especially the loss of your prior self-expectations. Are they challenges or adventures? How might you react emotionally? How do you hope to react? What are you going to do when problems arise? Are you going to choose adaptive coping strategies?

What are you going to do now to take control back and prevent problems from snowballing? What is most important to you? Can you be more flexible with your life and expectations? Are you showing yourself compassion? Are you continuing to build and feed your social network? How do you resist the social isolation that too commonly occurs with aging? There are many things that people have done to maintain and grow more resilient as they age.

What You Can Do for Yourself

- Dedicate time and energy to a worthy cause.
    - This increases flexibility of thinking and puts your attention on something greater than yourself.
- Celebrate small wins.
- Learn something new—online course, learn to play the guitar, and so on.
    - This also increases flexibility of thinking and refocuses your attention if you are having maladaptive thoughts.
- Ask what you can change about your situation and ask positively.
    - Even prisoners of war, who suffered greatly, were able to find areas of growth and meaning in their lives when they focused on what they could change or do with their situation.
- How can you stay grounded in the present moment? Adapt your behavior. Hang on to what is most important in your life.
- Make a list of your skills and focus on your strengths.
    - Include even the smallest things (e.g., kindness, love animals, be an avid reader, haven't gotten a ticket, I can bake a yummy pie, etc.).
- Describe someone in your life who has been resilient that you admire.
- Write or record stories of your life for the next generations.
- Take a creative risk without fear of making a mistake.
    - Laugh at mistakes and enjoy them as opportunities (growth mindset).
- Listen to music and sing out loud.

- Write in a journal daily, including not only what you did but reactions and emotions.
- Finding ways to connect with others.
    - It may be as simple as saying "Hi" to the pharmacist or asking the checkout person at the grocery store about their day.
- Practice finding words to express your emotions.
- Exercise and eat healthy to build confidence and ability.
- Seek help from professionals, psychiatrists, psychologists, therapists, religious leaders, and life coaches.

Have a Plan

My father-in-law is seventy-six years old, and we went hiking with him today, with his two granddogs at our heels. He kept up a shockingly fast pace for six miles, faster than the lab-shepherd mix! He just retired less than a year ago, and we didn't know what he was going to do. We worried because he is a quiet, humble man, and work seemed all-encompassing, and it provided his social outlet as well. He had a plan. Now he spends more time camping and fishing. He hikes every day and studies the behavior of the wildlife—elk, deer, mountain lions, owls, and bald eagles—in the meadows behind his home. He's made new friends with some of the neighbors and is making plans for future road trips with and to see his sister. He is happy and carefree.

Another patient of mine is a surgeon who, due to illness, can no longer perform operations. His mind remains sharp, and he still has something to offer. He can still see patients in the office and decide who needs surgery and who doesn't. He volunteers on a remote Native American reservation that doesn't have surgeons where he is able to treat many and to help make arrangements for those who need surgery to be transported to the closest city for care. He is providing a great service. Instead of hanging up his shingle for good, he found a way to put his skills towards a worthy and much-needed cause.

I've seen others who have been asked to be resilient so many times in their life that they give up out of pure fatigue of will. If you are there, how might you be rescued from this exhaustion? What keeps you going? What gives you resilience? What allows you to dig deep and hold on in the most difficult moments so that we can get you to the practices mentioned above? Let your doctor know so that they can help.

It is not always apparent when one needs support to be resilient. If you want to go it alone, okay. But I would recommend that you reach out and ask for a hand. There are many people willing and able to help. There are certainly many in the same boat who would love if you could team up and help keep each other afloat.

CHAPTER TWENTY-FOUR
ADVANCE DIRECTIVES: YOU HAVE A SAY OVER YOUR LIFE

A Good Death

I think it is fair to say that everything I learned about palliative care, hospice, and advance directives I learned from dear friends and career-long colleagues Jeanie Youngwerth, MD, and Harri Brackett, RN, CNS, ACHPN, who practice Hospice and Palliative Care at the University of Colorado. I appreciate them both as the three of us share common values around the need to maintain dignity and humanity through aging, advanced illness, and the dying process. That is why we take on difficult topics with our patients and are willing to have hard conversations. We also feel strongly that *merely having completed an advance directive is not enough.*

For years, I worked in the hospital, spending a majority of my time on the geriatric inpatient ward of the UCHealth University of Colorado Hospital. I witnessed good deaths and bad deaths. Yes, you heard me correctly. There is such a thing as a good death.

Some people are not afraid to think about death and, in fact, look for others to talk to about their hopes and fears. Many patients wanted to talk to me about death because every time they mentioned the topic to family, they received silencing comments such as, "Don't talk like that," "You are doing great," or "You have many more years to live!" Others have been afraid of dying since they were young children and find the topic hard to broach. Either way, it is so important to find the inner strength, time, and space to have these conversations so that others know what a good death means to you.

For some, a good death means dying at home surrounded by loved ones, free of pain and suffering, listening to their favorite music, or having their cat or dog in bed with them. For others, a good death means dying in a nursing home where their family is not burdened by having to take care of them but can be at their side solely for the purposes of enjoying spending time with them. They, too, wish to be free of pain and suffering. For the rare few, they prefer to die away from their families so as to completely unburden their loved ones from the trauma of witnessing their death. And then there are some that like to go down fighting, even if that means dying in a hospital alone connected to machines, tubes, and wires, unable to communicate with those around them.

To me, a bad death occurs when doctors and families don't know what a patient wants and feel legally obligated or so morally conflicted that they choose to "do everything." As a result, I have seen needless, long-lasting pain and recurrent suffering inflicted on patients that neither improves the quality of their lives nor extends the length of their life. Such unfortunate circumstances are heartbreaking for all and cause unimaginable and often unrecognized trauma in family members, their bedside nurses, and health-care teams. To this, I bear witness.

Definition of Advance Directives

Advance directive is a generic umbrella term that includes various documents and designations that ensure you get the type of medical care that you want when you are not able to speak for yourself. Most patients associate advance directives with catastrophic illness or injury and delay getting them until they are "older." In truth, every adult needs them. As a doctor, I rely on them all the time, even for mildly ill patients. What if you experience a medication side effect and become confused? You may be otherwise healthy but can no longer speak for yourself. I had a healthy middle-aged woman accidentally take her husband's medication instead of her vitamins and end up confused. She needed to be treated with reversal medication, but we needed consent to do so. We recently had a patient who fell off his bicycle, struck his face, and broke his jaw. Between his swollen eyes and inability to speak clearly, I needed someone else to help with consent forms so that he could get the treatment he needed. It would have been easier if he had advance directives completed.

Types of Advance Directives

Advance directives guide both the kinds of healthcare that you do and do not want and who can speak on your behalf if you are unable. Types of advance directives include:

- A living will
- A medical durable power of attorney
- A medical proxy
- Code status document

Let's take a look at them each more closely and discuss how they are used by doctors, patients, and families. The living will was designed to alert medical professionals and your family to the medical treatments that you would or wouldn't want to receive. It often includes whether or not you would want treatments such as mechanical ventilation (a breathing machine via a tube in your throat), artificial nutrition (through a tube up your nose or through a hole cut in your abdomen), ICU care, IV antibiotics, or blood transfusions. Most living wills tie these treatments to very specific scenarios. For example, "If I was in a vegetative state, I would not want to receive artificial nutrition." They might even state for how long you would want to receive treatment: "I do not want to be on a ventilator for more than seven days."

How Do Doctors Use Living Wills?

Practically speaking, *doctors don't use living wills.* Unfortunately, physicians find the living will documents to be very unhelpful as the scenarios documented in the living wills are so rare that they almost never apply to the patient's current medical situation. Therefore, they can't be used by doctors to guide medical decision-making. The other problem is that when a patient is unable to speak for themselves, it is often an emergency. In emergencies, the living will is never available, and even if it is, the doctor doesn't have time to read it as he or she needs to be tending to the patient.

Instead, they *rely completely on the patient's medical durable power of attorney* to make medical decisions. A medical durable power of attorney makes medical decisions for you when you are unable. The living will does help a person start to think about what they would or would not want for their future, and it helps facilitate discussions with their medical durable power of attorney. A medical durable power of attorney or medical proxy makes medical decisions for you when you are unable.

If you don't legally appoint a person to be your medical durable power of attorney to speak on your behalf, in most states, you may verbally appoint someone to be your medical proxy (also called a healthcare proxy) to make decisions for you. You can only appoint someone if you have capacity. Capacity requires that you have the mental capacity to understand your circumstances, consider risks and benefits of treatment, weigh them against a belief system, and communicate your wishes in a clear and consistent manner. Then the proxy would step in when you no longer meet the criteria for capacity. For example, you might appoint your brother to be your medical proxy before your colonoscopy. You are allowed to make all of your medical decisions until you get anesthesia; then, since you can no longer speak for yourself while under anesthesia, your brother is now in charge.

If you do not designate a medical durable power of attorney or a medical proxy, then a medical proxy is appointed to speak on your behalf if you can't speak for yourself. If you have an unexpected accident or illness, do not have capacity, and you have not designated anyone, the laws of the state decide who will be your medical proxy. For example, the laws in Colorado are complicated and not clear. In some states, the spouse automatically becomes the medical proxy . . . not in Colorado. In Colorado, all "interested parties" gather, and together, they decide who will be the decision maker for you, and that person becomes your sole decision maker. "Interested parties" could be family, friends, neighbors, co-workers, or anyone who knows and voices care for you. Because the law is so vague and may vary depending on where you find yourself, I would encourage you to designate someone and officially appoint them as your medical durable power of attorney or at least your medical proxy. Your "interested parties" may pick someone who doesn't know you well or imposes their values and wishes that are very different from yours.

How Do You Pick a Medical Durable Power of Attorney or Proxy?

Who should you pick? Most people pick their spouse. I didn't. For me, my spouse would have a very hard time letting go . . . which is in accordance with my wishes. She would also be emotionally traumatized forever. Thus, I chose a friend who could be available that cares but could also be more objective. For me, I actually think this decision is in my family's and friend's best interest.

It is crucially important for the person who you want to make decisions on your behalf to know you, your beliefs, and what is important to you. The living will won't have the answers they are seeking, but if they know what you want, then that person won't be burdened by the decisions that they are asked to make. For some, life is not worth living if they can't read and write; for others, it is not worth living if they are reliant on others for toileting, while others feel that life is always worth living. Tell your decision maker what makes life worth living for you.

You should also make sure they have an active list of your medications, medical history, surgical history, and allergies, as well as the name and phone number of your primary care doctor. They should be ready to provide this to any healthcare professional if you are unable to do so yourself.

Make the Conversation Easier

Some people find these conversations very difficult to initiate with family members and with the person they want to be their medical proxy in part because they find potential scenarios impossible to imagine. For example, you may not want to be on a breathing machine for pneumonia because you have bad lungs and don't want to have to recover from another severe pneumonia, but what if you got stung on the lip by a bumblebee and only needed to be on the machine for twelve hours until the swelling went down? There are websites that provide tools to facilitate discussions. They are all different, and one is not better than the other:

- theconversationproject.org
- prepareforyourcare.org
- med.stanford.edu/letter.html
- getyourshittogether.org

There is even a card game called Go Wish (available at www.gowish.org) that can facilitate discussions.

CPR

The last piece of the advance directive is the CPR directive, and that is state-specific. The CPR directive refers only to your code status. Code status refers to what you want a medical professional to do when you die: Would you like them to attempt to bring you back to life (full code), or would you like them to allow you to have a natural death (DNR or DNAR)? DNAR stands for "do not attempt resuscitation" and has replaced the term DNR (do not resuscitate) since resuscitation is rarely successful. If you are a full code, when you die, healthcare professionals will proceed with CPR—chest compressions, place a tube in your throat, and, if you regain a pulse, connect you to a ventilator or breathing machine. The overall survival to hospital discharge after CPR for all ages is about 15 percent (and not all 15 percent go home; many end up in a nursing home and with brain damage). When deciding on code status, it is important for patients over eighty years old and those with metastatic cancer to know that, if they were to die and receive CPR, the chance of returning home and having a functional life is close to nil. I tell you this because I think most people are not adequately informed when they are deciding on their code status, and having information helps them feel most secure in their decisions.

My Favorite Documents

The Five Wishes is a living will that is the most patient-, family-, and physician-friendly version of a will that I have ever found. I particularly like it because it is written in simple, practical language and extends beyond medical procedures. It is also valid in most states in the United States and can be purchased online for $5.

Most states have their own medical proxy forms and CPR directive forms that you can download off the Internet for free.

Completing these documents can be overwhelming, but your doctor should gladly help you. There is one more document that you may see called the MOST form, which I personally use for sicker patients. The

MOST form should always be filled out with a physician and with a thorough discussion.

Common Patient Questions

I have been asked a few questions from patients in the past that you might have as well. One patient asked, "What happens if the ambulance takes you to a hospital you know will not honor your wishes due to their religious dicta and/or if you are just not comfortable with the level of care at that hospital?" While this is a scary prospect, it does happen. There are some religious hospitals that will have hospital policies that supersede your wishes. For example, no matter how much you beg and plead with the local Catholic hospital, they aren't going to provide contraception. Likewise, say your proxy conveys your wishes to be removed from a breathing machine or to have artificial nutrition stopped if you haven't shown any signs of improvement. Some religious hospitals may continue treatment based on their values regardless of your wishes. If you did end up in such a hospital, you could request a transfer to another hospital. This is more easily done from the emergency room prior to admission, but it is possible. Be persistent if the wishes of the person you represent are not being honored. A medical durable power of attorney is much more effective in these situations than a medical proxy. The hospital you are leaving is responsible for accommodating travel and transfer to the new hospital. The patient, however, must be clinically stable . . . meaning they won't die during the transportation from one hospital to another.

Another popular question is, "Do DNR tattoos work?" Unfortunately, they do not. It is not that simple. Patients need to have capacity to make their own healthcare decisions, meaning they must be able to communicate at a basic level their understanding of the medical situation, consider the risks and benefits of treatment options, weigh it against their values, and communicate their wishes while not suffering from a debilitating mental health problem like depression that could cloud their judgment. There is no way to assess a patient's capacity when they got the tattoo. Also, patients are allowed to change their mind and sometimes do so based on the situation that arises.

Let me give you a sad example: One of my patients with intermittent episodes of depression, in a moment of deep sadness, decided to overdose on medication. Just prior to swallowing all of his pills, he wrote DNR on his chest. He was revived, hospitalized first medically and then psychiatrically. Two months later, his depression had passed, and he was so grateful to have survived. This is just one example of why DNR tattoos don't and shouldn't work.

Palliative Care and Hospice Are Different

Slightly tangential to the topic of advance directives, but I also want to mention palliative care and hospice because many people confuse the two. I think this is a very important distinction to make. Palliative care is a group of doctors and medical staff that are dedicated to taking care of patients with advanced disease. They focus on your quality of life to ensure that your medical treatment plan addresses and relieves unpleasant symptoms like pain, constipation, and shortness of breath while ensuring that you have the best possible support to participate in activities that are meaningful to you. Palliative care is provided *alongside* curative or otherwise active treatment of chronic illnesses.

Hospice also provides relief from unwanted symptoms and provides support to you as a whole person, but it is for people who are at the end of their lives. Hospice prioritizes comfort *rather than* treating disease for the purposes of curing or extending life. To be clear, when a patient enters hospice, many of their medications are stopped, and only medications that bring comfort are continued, and they no longer go to the hospital or have procedures. Every medication and intervention offered are only for the purpose of making the patient comfortable. However, people who engage with either palliative or hospice care often live longer and have an improved quality of life. These are resources that your doctor may not readily offer. You may have to ask your doctor to provide a referral to speak with a palliative care or hospice team to learn more about what they can offer you.

What You Can Do for Yourself

- Consider what a good death looks like to you.
- Order the Five Wishes form online and fill it out.
- Identify someone to make medical decisions on your behalf if you are ever unable.

- Pick one or two tools listed above to talk with them about what is important to you (e.g., having everything done and living as long as possible, only living if you can communicate, not dying in the hospital, etc.).
- Decide on a code status with that medical decision maker.
- If you are faced with a serious diagnosis, ask your doctor lots of questions, such as the following:
    - "What will happen if we pursue {plan A} versus {plan B} versus only treating the symptoms? What should I expect from each option?"
    - Ask the hard questions: ask about pain, quality of life, length of life, cost, housing, nursing care, and independence.
    - If a doctor avoids answering, ask another doctor. Some doctors are more up-front about negative possible outcomes. Some doctors are more comfortable talking about the end of life.
- If you think you might benefit from palliative care or hospice, ask your physician for a referral.
- Talk to your faith community if you are struggling with decisions.

What Can Your Doctor Do?

- Match your medical treatment plan with who you are as an individual and with your priorities in life
- Help you predict the likely medical complications you will endure and help you anticipate how they will affect every aspect of your life
- Answer your questions about life-sustaining measures
- Provide referrals to palliative care and hospice teams

Dying Is a Process

I teach my students and residents that just like birth is a nine-month process, death is also a process. Often, patients seek medical attention while they are in the process of dying, and we do everything we can to treat their health problems when, in fact, we put them in a state of death limbo.

Unlike years ago, bodies can be kept alive on machines for a while or even for indefinite periods of time. We have machines that can mechanically squeeze the heart, replace the kidneys, breathe for us, infuse nutrition into our veins, and so on. As death looms, life can eventually become a painful existence with questionable purpose once the body can no longer communicate with the world and the brain loses function. Families need guidance to know how to proceed and when to say enough is enough. These decisions are very difficult for family members, medical durable powers of attorney, and proxies. They are often asked to withhold or withdraw treatment.

Withdrawing versus Withholding Treatment

Withdrawing treatment refers to stopping treatment, such as IV fluids or artificial nutrition, while withholding treatment means never starting it in the first place. Withdrawing treatment is infinitely more difficult for family members and medical decision makers than to never have started it in the first place. Both are easier if your decision maker knows what you want. No one wants to have to guess what their loved one would want under the pressure of an emergency situation. Please do your power of attorney and medical proxy a favor and provide them guidance so that they can follow your wishes with less internal conflict.

Medical Aid in Dying

Some states even offer programs that allow patients to choose the timing of their deaths. Terminally ill adults may request a prescription from their doctor for medications that will bring about a peaceful death. There is a very specific process to ensure that the patient requesting medical aid in dying is mentally capable, has a prognosis of six months or less, and is sure about their decision. The treatment affords dying people control and compassion during a very difficult period of their lives. Currently, medical aid in dying is available in California, Colorado, District of Columbia, Hawaii, Maine, Montana, New Jersey, Oregon, Vermont, and Washington.

You Decide

The powerful message here is that most people have choice over their final days! Because doctors can anticipate death most of the time, you can help plan what you want for the end of your life in advance. For you and the people you care about, take the steps now to plan for the future. The difficult conversations now will bring much peace of mind in the future. I guarantee it.

CHAPTER TWENTY-FIVE
HOME SAFETY: ON THE SAME LEVEL

Take a Look Around

At thirty-eight years old, we searched for what I hoped would be the home we would live in for the rest of our lives. As we toured homes with our realtor, I looked to make sure that there was a bedroom and full bathroom on the ground floor. I checked to see if there was enough room to cover the entryway steps with a ramp. Yes, the bathroom tub could be replaced with a walk-in shower, and there was room to eventually move the washer and dryer up to the ground floor from the basement if needed. The realtor looked at me curiously, with my thirty-eight-year-old energy and enthusiasm and asked, "Jeannette, who did you say is going to be living in this house?" I grinned and said, "We are! But you see, I'm a geriatrician, and it's got to last the duration!"

One of the benefits of doing home visits is that I get to see how my patients live and if their homes are as safe as they can be. It was Benjamin Franklin who said, "An ounce of prevention is worth a pound of cure." The first part of the home visit is always trying to find where my patients live. Given the complexity of some of these housing developments, I am convinced that my patients are testing to see how smart their doctor is!

Once I successfully find their homes, I frequently find my patients surrounded by others—spouses, children, grandchildren, caregivers, physical therapists, visiting clergy, housekeepers, or no one. This information is very important as it gives me some idea of the level of support that the patient has or may need. I then meet with my patient. We get caught up on interim events since the last appointment and follow up on new and chronic health problems. I check their vital signs, complete a physical exam, draw blood, and place orders. Then we talk about home safety as they give me a tour of the home. I ask patients to show me where they like to sit or spend most of their day, where their bathroom is, where they sleep, and the location of their kitchen.

I also ask patients to show me their medications. For a doctor, this is always the scariest and most valuable part. On quite a few instances, I have had patients open up a nightstand with thousands of loose unlabeled pills of all shapes, sizes, and colors, saying, "I take these every day, just like you tell me." Usually, I am handed a reused plastic grocery bag full of pill bottles, containing their current medications, as well as multiple bottles of the same medication and old bottles of medications they are no longer supposed to be taking. At this point, I begin combining like medications and separating out medications no longer prescribed, placing a big "X" on the label. Other times, my anxieties are relieved by a stack of neatly organized bottles and a properly filled pillbox with the correct number of pills obviously taken for the week.

By way of sharing everything I have learned, I'm going to provide you with a list of things that you can do to make your house safer as you age.

What You Can Do for Yourself

- Medication errors are one of the leading causes of death in America. Organize your medications or have someone help you organize your medication if that is not one of your strengths.
    - On each pill bottle, write what the medication is for. For example, on the bottle of lisinopril, write "high blood pressure."
    - If you are supposed to stop a medication, put a big X on the bottle with the date, and store the bottle separate from the medications you need to take every day.
    - If you have multiple pills of the same kind and the same dose, combine them into one bottle.

   - Buy a pillbox with rows for when you need to take your medications. For example, if you take your medications in the morning and at night, the pillbox should have two rows, with seven boxes for each day of the week in each row. Or try out the automatic pillboxes that connect to phone apps and open different doors when it's time to take your medication.
   - Fill the pillbox regularly.
- Falls are a leading cause of injury in seniors.
   - Remove throw rugs.
   - Remove wheels from chairs.
   - Clean up piles of clutter.
   - Widen walkways and paths to at least thirty-two inches across, even if you have to donate furniture to make more room to move around.
   - Move electrical cords out of the way and consider affixing them to the moldings.
   - Wear nonstick footwear that is secure on your feet.
   - Do you have a cane or walker that you are willing and able to use? In Colorado, many older people use hiking poles instead of canes because it makes them feel younger; others find hiking poles more comfortable on the wrist than a standard cane or walker.
   - Install railings on both sides of all stairs, inside and outside of the home.
   - Placing different colors of duct tape along the edge of each stair step can help seniors see the steps better. Consider adding nonstick treads on steps too.
   - Some may need stairlifts installed.
- Renovate the bathroom as it is the most dangerous room in the house.
   - Install grab bars in the shower or tub area and beside the toilet.
   - Consider elevating the toilet seat. Make sure that your feet can still touch the ground when you sit. You need to have your feet firmly on the ground to engage the abdominal

muscles to have a bowel movement (this is why toddlers struggle to poop—their feet are dangling).
    - Roll out the rubber mat and place it in the tub to prevent slipping.
    - Consider a shower chair and handheld showerhead.
    - Set the thermostat on the water heater to less than 120 degrees Fahrenheit to prevent accidental burns.
    - Install a nightlight in the bathroom and everywhere else. I like the LED motion detector lights by General Electric.
    - You may need to install a walk-in shower, rather than one where you have to step into a tub. Extended shower chairs can help you slide into a tub without having to step over the tub while standing.
- Decorate the refrigerator.
    - List 911, emergency contacts, family members' phone numbers, the patient's primary care doctor, and poison control (1-800-222-1222), and place these numbers on the refrigerator.
    - Place a copy of your CPR directive and medical durable power of attorney's name and phone number on the refrigerator. Paramedics know to look there for instruction.
- Simplify technology.
    - Make sure you have a phone that you can use.
    - Ideally, a phone that can be kept in the pocket will keep you from feeling like you have to run to pick up the phone.
    - Enlarge the font or find someone who can help you . . . just do what I do, and ask the youngest person in the room. Even the eight-year-olds are better at programming the phones than I am.
    - Ensure that you can easily call family members and know when they are calling.
- Protect against fire.
    - Change the batteries in your smoke detectors and carbon monoxide detectors on New Year's Day and the Fourth of July.
    - Check for damaged or frayed electrical cords or overloaded power strips.

  - Remove candles and space heaters from the home.
  - If dementia sets in, unplug stoves or have them disconnected from the gas line.
- Make the kitchen friendlier.
  - Unclutter the cabinets and rearrange items to limit reaching and bending.
  - Install pullout shelves in cabinets for easier access.
  - If possible, use a refrigerator with a lower drawer freezer.
  - Elevate the front of the refrigerator so that the door always closes.
  - Install a swivel plate into the corner cabinets to avoid bending and reaching.
  - Use an electric teakettle that automatically shuts off rather than a stovetop kettle.
  - Consider color coding the hot faucet with a red rubberized water faucet cover and the cold with a blue rubberized water faucet cover.
  - Replace round kitchen water faucets with levers.
  - Clean out the refrigerator and food cupboard or pantry weekly. Throw out expired and soured food.
- The monsters aren't under the bed.
  - The monster *is* the bed. It can be really hard to get out of a sagging soft mattress. Replace it with a firm one that is at a height that will allow you to get in and out of easily but that is not so high as to cause injury if you were to fall out.
  - I've seen some great floor-to-ceiling telescoping grab bars beside the bed to help seniors get in and out of bed.
  - Keep a flashlight near the bed . . . just in case there *are* monsters under the bed.
  - Keep a sturdy chair in the bedroom for dressing.
- More home renovation projects.
  - Replace round doorknobs with levers instead.
  - Replace burnt-out light bulbs and install more light fixtures.
  - You may need to move light switches.
  - Remove locks from inside doors.
  - Keep stairs and paths clean of snow, ice, and leaf debris or hire a service or neighbor to help.

- You may need to widen doorways.
- Research alert necklaces and bracelets.

What Your Doctor Can Do

- Home visits are too rare these days. If your doctor doesn't do home visits, you can ask him or her for a home safety evaluation, which is usually performed by a nurse or occupational therapist. They can assess your living situation and see if there are any dangers that you might have overlooked and help you think through how to remedy the situation.

Simple Fixes

Of all of the things that I do as a doctor, home visits are the most time-consuming, yet I don't mind. They are the most valuable thing that I do. Mr. Jones kept falling and hitting his head in the bathroom. He didn't want to do any major construction on his home, but when he showed me his bathroom, we were able to find armrests for the toilet that would not require drilling into the floors or walls. He hasn't fallen since, and we didn't disrupt his home.

Mrs. Cohen, who has mild dementia, was plagued with perpetually uncontrolled blood pressure. The first visit, she showed me her drawer of loose pills. (AAAHHH!!!) The second visit, I had her show me the pill bottles that had been delivered. She was missing her amlodipine. Her daughter delivered amlodipine from the pharmacy, and on the third visit, I brought a pillbox to her house. Now she fills it every week, her blood pressure is at goal, and we have an amazing doctor-patient relationship, because I have grown to truly know her and her daughter at these extended visits. For other patients, I have arranged for a nurse to go to their homes weekly to fill their pillboxes, as this is usually covered by insurance.

These home visits truly let me understand how I can best help each individual senior patient. I can now provide more specific recommendations tailored to what each person needs, can do, is able to afford, and what practically works for him or her and their families, so that he or she can have a long, healthy, happy, injury-free, and independent life.

CHAPTER TWENTY-SIX
ELDER ABUSE: LOOK OUT FOR EACH OTHER

Myths and Misconceptions

There are a lot of misconceptions about elder abuse.

1. Myth—Abuse only occurs when someone hits another person.
   When it comes to the elderly, abuse also includes sexual abuse, emotional abuse, neglect, abandonment, and financial neglect and exploitation.
2. Myth—Most elder abuse occurs in nursing homes.
   Most elder abuse occurs in one's home.
3. Myth—Most elder abuse is perpetrated by a stranger.
   I wish this were true, but unfortunately, most elders are abused by family members, making the betrayal more devastating.
4. Myth—If a person denies abuse, it isn't happening.
   Many victims deny abuse for fear of the consequences of confronting the abuser, fear how their living situation might change, or because they don't remember.
5. Myth—It won't happen to me because . . . (fill in the blank).
   Everyone says that, until it does.

CHAPTER TWENTY-SIX

Types of Elder Abuse

If you saw a friend walking over a patch of ice, would you warn them of the danger and reach out an arm to guide them? Seniors protect seniors all of the time. This is another area in which we need to understand the dangers so that we can keep on the lookout for our friends and family. We need to protect each other. Here's what you need to know:

- Physical abuse—Someone causes bodily harm to another. This could even include restraining the elderly, tying them to furniture, or locking them in a room.
- Emotional abuse—This occurs when the patient is subjected to painful words, yelling, threats, or isolation from others.
- Neglect—Some older adults are denied food, medication, and access to health care or other basic needs.
- Abandonment—This occurs when an older adult who can't take care of themselves is left alone without a plan of care, either at home or at a hospital or in a public place. If an elderly person can recognize emergencies, call 911, and communicate an emergency, they probably are safe to be left alone.
- Sexual abuse—Forced participation in or being forced to watch sexual acts is sexual abuse.
- Financial neglect—This happens when a patient is no longer able to pay their bills and responsible adults do not help.
- Financial exploitation—Many elderly people are exploited for their money without their consent, under false pretenses or through manipulation. Theft of personal items also occurs.

Signs of Abuse and Neglect

According to the National Institutes of Health (NIH) and the Centers for Disease Control and Prevention (CDC), we need to be most protective of our friends and family with memory problems and those who are socially isolated. Here are some signs of abuse and neglect.

- Your loved one or friend stops taking part in activities.
- Looks disheveled with lack of basic hygiene.

- Lacks clean clothing or weather-appropriate clothing.
- Has changes in sleep patterns.
- Unexpected weight loss.
- Behavioral changes, including becoming more withdrawn or agitated.
- Unexplained bruises, burns, cuts, and/or scars.
- Bedsores.
- Evictions or lack of working utilities.
- Lack of food in the house.
- Unclean or overly cluttered living conditions.
- Home in need of repair or that presents fire or other safety hazards.
- Unusual spending patterns.
- A new best friend accepting "gifts."
- An elder's life circumstances don't match their financial assets.
- Signatures on checks that don't match.
- Large withdrawals from bank accounts.
- Apparent lack of medical care or medical aids like walkers, glasses, hearing aids, and/or medications.

How Do You Prevent Elder Abuse Before It Starts?

How wonderful it would be if all abuse could be prevented before it starts, or at least caught early. There are certainly things that we can safeguard each other against as we age together.

What You Can Do for Others

- Listen to older adults and their caregivers to understand their challenges and provide support.
- Report abuse or suspected abuse to Adult Protective Services or their doctor.
- Check in often on your aging friends and family.
- Encourage elders to attend community events.
- Make sure everyone in your community stays active.
- Provide overburdened caregivers with support.

- Encourage caregivers to attend support groups.
- Inform others of any solicitations they should be aware of.
- Encourage friends to:
    - Seek professional help for drug, alcohol, and depression concerns and urge caregivers to do the same.
    - Be selective when choosing caregivers or help your friends pick caregivers.
    - Post and open their own mail and be aware of their own finances.
    - Shred documents with personal information and old credit cards.
    - Keep a close eye on credit card statements for fraudulent charges.
    - Never give personal information over the phone, by mail, or over the Internet unless you know the receiver.
    - Directly deposit all checks.
    - Have their own phone.
    - Review their will.
    - Install quality monitoring systems and consider a dog for security (my personal bias).
    - Make sure that their home is well lit at night.
    - Know their neighbors.
    - Lock their windows and doors.
    - Close their garage door before they go out.
    - Not accept help from strangers at their home.
    - Use a safe for valuables and important paperwork.
    - Keep valuables out of plain sight.

Reporting known or suspected abuse may be one of the hardest decisions that you have ever had to make. If calling Adult Protective Services is too difficult for you, then at least notify your friend's or family member's doctor. Let them know of your concerns. They likely have more information about the person's medical and social situation to add that can help determine the severity of the situation. While the doctor may not be able to release specific information about their patient, they can guide you and work with you to provide the means for addressing your concerns and the situation. They may even offer to unburden you and handle the situation themselves.

What If It Happens to You?

Elder abuse is common. If you suspect that you have been a victim, don't be ashamed.

Con artists are good, and they fool people of all ages. Every state and community has an elder abuse hotline that can provide guidance and education about the resources available for help in your community. Your physician, as well, can help. I have made both anonymous and non-anonymous calls on behalf of patients to gather information, understand the resources available, and troubleshoot possible paths to pursue so that patients could decide how they wanted to move forward.

In terms of resources, you should also know that most communities also have Respite Care available to provide relief for overburdened and stressed caregivers. Respite Care will provide care for a dependent elder, so that the caregiver can get a break for an afternoon, several days, or a few weeks.

There are times in all of our lives where we feel like we have lost control, but that doesn't mean you can't get it back. This can lead to feelings of anger, shame, despair, sadness, and grief. Remember, doctors don't just treat disease. We treat people. We care for people of all ages, including the elderly that have suffered from abuse. You may also have friends that can help, but I know not everyone has friends, and sometimes, professional experience can be more helpful. Reach out and find someone to help you get control of your life back. As long as you are alive, there is always time to get back on your feet and change the direction of the train. Then you will have an even better perspective to help a friend and protect your community.

There is no better cause than for a community to come together and advocate and support each other than over preventing elder abuse. It will bring you a sense of belonging, purpose, safety, and security. May you be united in looking out for one another.

CHAPTER TWENTY-SEVEN
ADAPTATION: MOUNTAINS TO CLIMB

My First Patient

We all age, but how we do it matters. Let me tell you about my first patient. Of course, I can't tell you his name. But, at the time, I can tell you that I had never known anyone with his name before but not because it was unique or from an unfamiliar ethnic community or race. If he had been a woman, his name would have been something like Edith, Hazel, or Mabel. It was a handsome, proud name, just unfamiliar, as names from prior generations can be. I was only twenty-one years old.

He and his family taught me many things. They taught me about levels of generosity to me, a stranger, that I had never seen or felt before. This first patient gave me courage and confidence to work with and learn from a body other than my own. I learned that our bodies talk in metaphors, and that despite having discrete organs, everything in our bodies is entirely connected. Perhaps, I always had empathy, but I grew to understand it and how important it was in being present in life and in connecting with others.

All I knew at first was his name, his date of birth, his height, his skin color, and the color of the remaining hairs on the top of his head. He had two tattoos—one of Poland, and one of Betty Boop in a sailor's uniform. I assumed that he had been a Navy veteran from World War II. I searched for his obituary and learned that he had died at eighty-six years old, was married for almost seventy years, and had a home full of children, grandchildren, and great-grandchildren every holiday.

There is another lesson, though, that I learned and I hope you will benefit from. As I learned from my first patient, my first cadaver in medical school. He had survived hip surgery, knee surgery, cholesterol plaque buildup in the arteries of his heart, the placement of three heart stents, a traumatic abdominal wound, removal of part of his colon, and a type of blood cancer that causes the spleen to enlarge to the size of a football. And those were only the diseases that I as a first-year medical student could identify. I'm sure there were many more. I remember being shocked at his body's physical resilience to endure so many diseases, injuries, and life stresses and to still persevere through each setback to the age of eighty-six.

My medical school was unique in that we got to know the name of our cadavers and also to meet their families at the end of the year to thank them. Believe it or not, I was a very shy young woman at that time and only hope now that I was able to convey my deepest appreciation and gratitude for their gift to my learning as a student and development as a human being.

I walked away from that experience thinking, on so many levels, "Fear not. You are stronger than you think!" And despite all of the changes that happen to the body over time, I hope that you, too, will remember that your body, mind, and soul are stronger than you think.

Learning to Adapt

Living in Colorado, I spend much of my free time hiking. Last weekend, I went with my spouse and our two dogs on one of our usual adventures. We donned our hiking boots, zip-off pants, several layers of shirts, and wind jackets. We lathered up with sunscreen, threw on hats, and leashed up the dogs. We put the lab-shepherd mix, which we fondly refer to as the leopard, into the trunk of the mini SUV. Truthfully, we just opened the gate, and she bounded in. The other small dog was secured in a crate on the back seat. We settled in the front seats. As we were trying to decide the best hiking trail for the day, I was reminded that the backpack with water, two sports bars, two apples, and two dog treats was still sitting on the kitchen table. (Senior moment?) By the time I had run back into the house, collected the pack, and returned to the car, the park's pass was dangling from the rearview mirror and a trail had been chosen.

We set off to a nearby state park, and forty minutes later, we were at the trailhead of a six-mile trail labeled, "Most difficult." Clearly, it was not of my choosing, but I've learned to pretend that this New Yorker is as tough as my surrounding Coloradoans. When I opened the passenger back door, my twenty-five-pound female Shiba Inu, Koi, slowly stood up, and I lifted her from the car to the pavement. Then she was set free to sniff at the end of the leash where the pavement met the dirt and mostly rock trail in the Rocky Mountains.

If you are not familiar with the breed, Shiba Inus are a Japanese breed, and she looks like a small Akita or, to many, a fox with a curly tail. Like all of the dog breed books warned me, she is independent, spirited, playful, and "of her own mind." Let me give you an example or three that hopefully won't make me sound like the crazy dog mom that I am. When she was three months old, she climbed over the dog gate, opened the hall closet, and climbed three shelves to find a toy to play with. She then made her way back to the floor with the toy, unwrapped it, and left the toy for another day. There were also the times (many, many) that she opened the sliding door to the bedroom closet only to unzip my gym bag, uncap my sports drink, and help herself to the remaining drink without spilling a drop.

I find her so difficult to explain in a few words. It seems as if only stories convey what it means to parent a Shiba Inu. You see, our lab-shepherd mix, Madonna, the blond beauty, lives to please us, listens to our commands, and eats any treat you give her. She is a real dog. This Koi is not uniquely special, except that she is her breed. I must offer her three different types of dog treats for her to inspect before she chooses the one she finds most suitable.

Now, you might be thinking, "Just offer her one treat, and either she eats it, or she doesn't. She isn't starving." And yes, I was that way, strict with the rules and the alpha of the pack . . . until she turned nine. At age nine, she developed a lump on her left back leg, which on dogs is referred to as a hock, right at the level of the knee. It didn't bother her, but it bothered me. Unfortunately, human medicine and vet medicine are all too similar, and I knew it was bad. She ended up having cancer, a grade II osteosarcoma. So, despite seventeen years of paying my student loan debt, I still sat with $160,000 of loans plus a mortgage and did what I promised myself I would never do for a dog; I paid for my fuzzy four-legged child to get very expensive cancer treatment.

We opted for radiation treatments to her hock rather than amputation because we, and presumably she, love to hike as a family. After weeks of being sedated and put on a breathing machine *every day* so that she could lie still for radiation, she developed a total-body rash from the pain medication. Then that rash got infected with staph, and it was not plain old staph but instead a multi-drug-resistant staph bacteria that I likely brought home from the hospital. This water-adverse dog tolerated thrice-weekly medicated baths to rid her body of a resistant staph that no antibiotics could treat (except IV amikacin). After three months of treatment, she was left with a permanently hairless left hock, which we bravely call her chicken leg, and her spry spirit had fully returned, and she was back to hiking ten miles per adventure up the Rocky Mountains at her usual lightning speed.

Three years later, at twelve years of age, we woke up to find her lethargic and uncharacteristically lying at the foot of our bed. She was unable to lift her head, and there were piles of vomit all over the house. (Sorry that I didn't spare you that detail.) Fortunately, we have flooring and not carpet! We rushed her to the vet worried that her cancer had returned as her liver was painful and swollen. In the car, we were emotionally trying to prepare ourselves to let her go, as we have with other pets before.

The Emergency Department vet greeted us with a smile! "I have great news! Yes, her liver is inflamed as you thought, but her cancer has not returned. She ruptured her gallbladder and needs emergency surgery. It will cost $5,000 to $10,000."

You know that you have picked the right spouse when you hear, "It's only money, dear. And this is what money is for."

So, as I, after twenty years of payments, still sat with $140,000 of student loan debt and a mortgage, I did what I promised myself I would never do . . . again. I sent my baby to the operating room on a Saturday. They were not able to do the procedure laparoscopically, so she was left with an abdominal incision from her ribs to her pelvis. This story, too, has a good ending. She was soon back on the trails as if nothing had happened and sooner than I've ever seen a human recover.

Well, today she is fourteen. She can't see as well, so no longer feels comfortable jumping onto the backseat and walking into her crate. I lift her into and out of the car. It's not her favorite moment of the day. Perhaps, she doesn't like the way I pick her up, but I suspect she misses her independence. We no longer hike ten miles. We hike four to six per adventure and try to find the coolest times of the day, as she is less tolerant of the heat. We also try to pick hikes that are not as steep. And we now let her set the pace, which is turtle slow on the uphill sections and moderately paced on the flat stretches and downhill. We set a new record last weekend. It was our slowest hike per mile ever. I watch closely for signs of pain or arthritis, swelling or an unsteady gait. She seems fine, and I know she will ask to go for a mountain climb again tomorrow.

She's learned to adapt. For me, adapting to meet her needs has been effortless. I wouldn't have it any other way. We still get to hike as a family. She is still happy. She lives in the moment. She doesn't complain that we do things differently than when she was younger. And being a Shiba Inu, she would complain if it bothered her in the form of a grunt, snort, or side eye. (I swear I'm not making these things up. Ask other Shiba Inu parents!) She is grateful for the hikes even if they are shorter distances, and she still wants to go, knowing that I have to help her in and out the car and occasionally up large boulders on the trail. Our new pace leaves more time for her and Madonna to sniff, for us to enjoy the view, to take too many photos, watch the birds, and identify the flowers. Her aging process has been a gift for all of us.

Every day, as a doctor who treats aging patients, many of whom are my age or older, I am constantly facing my future. In my midlife, I already know which joints will give me trouble as I age, how my health will affect my future, and what new diseases I am likely to acquire. But I also know what I can do to prevent challenges. I know that it is easier said than done. Some people just love to exercise. They are innately driven to wake up, put their sneakers on, and go for a run. Well, that isn't me. In truth, I don't like to exercise and feel completely overwhelmed at the gym. Yet, every day, I exercise, because I like the way it makes my body feel: flexible, limber, and strong. Exercise improves my mental focus, makes me want to eat healthier and drink more water, gives me more energy to get through the day, and makes me more optimistic. I don't have physical limitations (yet) that prevent me from doing the things I want to do or that prevent me from keeping up with my friends. My previously broken ankle may yell at me for days after a hike, but I can still hike. The discomfort isn't anything ice can't fix, and hiking is worth the benefits to the rest of my body.

Yes, doctors practice what they preach because we have seen suffering and we don't want it for ourselves. Most doctors fear suffering more than death. And yes, doctors teach because we want you to have a long life full of high-quality years, and most of all, we don't want anyone to suffer unnecessarily.

Despite all that I have seen, I have a lot of reasons to remain optimistic about the aging process. I am realistic to know that from time to time injury, illness, and loss will take a serious blow to your sense of self and add challenges to your life. You will experience anguish, anger, sadness, and grief. But you don't have to lose your power, your agency, or who you are to the illness. Sometimes, setbacks are preventable, some are treatable, and some are not. Those that are not require adapting. You have the strength and ability to adapt if you allow yourself the flexibility. You can still extract pleasure, joy, and great meaning from your life, and I would hate for you to miss any of it. As long as you are alive, there is still so much life left to live and there is still time to seize the day.

There are days that will require you to search for hope and courage from deep within and to put faith and belief in the future of medicine, science, and advances in medical technology. There are always new tests, new medications, new therapies, and clinical trials on the horizon. You may or may not live long enough to see them emerge, but whoever thought we would see a vaccine developed in less than a year!

Use your friends and family to help find your inner strengths and to motivate you to take care of yourself. There might be times that you are putting on a bit of a front to look better for them than you feel so that they worry less. That grace in your presentation is likely serving you as well. Your family and friends need you as much as you need them.

Be honest with yourself about your abilities and limitations so that you can tackle them head-on. If you overestimate your abilities, you will not be able to adapt appropriately and will end up with more injuries, missed diagnoses, and being sicker in the long run. I'm sure you can see how this would lead to more suffering. Denial can be a large impervious wall for some.

Let others help in ways that are supportive to you, and instead of succumbing to dependence, find ways to help them back. Perhaps it is as simple as saying thank you and being grateful. A kind word or gesture goes a long way. Maybe you take time to get to know who your caregivers are as people. I'm sure you also have helpful stories to share.

Take pride in eating healthy foods and exercising. When I think of healthy food, I think of whole foods as they come off the plant or animal rather than processed. For example, I'd rather eat a grape than grape juice or corn than a corn chip. It will make you feel so much better, I promise. As for exercise, you will likely lose some level of fitness with time. If not strength, then flexibility. Even if you can only move your hands, do it every day with joy and appreciation. What amazing things can you do with what you have and how can you hold on to those abilities?

Adapt to your new realities. If you can no longer play kickball with your great-grandchildren, then bounce a rubber ball. You will still be creating lasting memories that can be passed down generation to generation.

Remain a participant of the world around you as you still can make vital contributions to the world. Be a friend, a neighbor, a religious participant, a community voice, a political voice, aware of the current news, etc.

Find a therapist or a coach to get you through the toughest times and provide a contained place to vent so that you both have an outlet to release your tensions and don't project unintentionally on those who care for you most.

Now, let me tell you about my grandfather. He loved to run, and he did so on the beach, no less! He was remarkably healthy into his late eighties, with no health problems and on no medications. One March, he caught pneumonia running in the cold wind. Grandma was very worried about losing him, so she made a rule that he could not run along the beach in the winter but had to run either indoors or on the neighborhood streets instead. He had to adapt. How did he adapt? He learned to wake up before she did, so that he could get in his winter morning beach runs before she noticed. And he would always return with breakfast, which he delivered to her with a secretly knowing smile!

CHAPTER TWENTY-EIGHT
CONCLUSION: YOU HAVE MORE LIFE TO LIVE

My Dad

Let me tell you about my dad. For as long as I can remember, he has been bald, just like all of his brothers. Decades later . . . not much has changed in that regard. He is as adorable as ever. Age, though, has presented a series of challenges or, as I prefer to call them, unexpected health adventures. In his early forties, he was diagnosed with a lifelong disease called sarcoidosis that causes abnormal cells to infiltrate your organs. His lungs, kidney, and heart have been affected. He has endured multiple cancers, including recurrences of two of them, and their less-than-pleasant treatments with accompanying disappointing and permanent side effects. And the list of health problems goes on.

Having worked at a hardware store and then a millwork company for his entire working life, he was lucky enough to have health insurance for most of his life, which afforded him access to healthcare. He worked with his doctors to treat and manage his health problems, maintained a normal weight, and ate a healthy diet, thanks to my mom's cooking and despite his persistent sweet tooth.

As a retiree, he has the benefit of Medicare, access to healthcare, still fits into his National Guard uniform from the 1960s, and has learned to sneak spoons of ice cream from the freezer after eating mom's healthy dinners. He has many accomplishments for which he is proud. One of those is his half-acre lawn. No, it is not the most beautifully manicured, nor is it free of weeds. He is proud that after living in the same house for seventy years, he can still mow the entire lawn with his push mower and that every autumn he (and my mom together) can continue to hand rake and bag over one hundred bags of leaves and acorns that have fallen from the numerous great old oak trees in their yard.

This year, he was awarded a Lifetime Achievement Award from the local fire department for over fifty years of active volunteer service to the department. His next goal is to make it to fifty-five years of active duty. While he no longer climbs on the tops of burning houses and buildings, he can still move around wearing thirty pounds of firefighter's gear with an additional thirty-pound tank of air on his back. He can still haul firehoses, open fire hydrants, and drive a firetruck.

Yes, aging has its adventures, but how lucky for the young firefighters on the squad to have someone around who has seen it all and can serve as a leader and mentor. In this role alone, age brings knowledge, experience, a sense of calm during emergencies, and the notion of what it means to be a professional and to truly be a dedicated member of the community.

My dad is not unique. He is not a Superman . . . except to me. I remember when he was first diagnosed with sarcoidosis, and he felt that his body had betrayed him. It was perhaps the first time he had to confront his mortality and loosen the illusion of being in total control of his body. He wasn't and is not always in control of his body, but he is and has always been in control of his life. He does the best he can to take care of himself, and he makes the most of every moment.

Never Lose Hope

Having had migraines since I was a child, I never experienced that "moment of betrayal." My body and I have long been at war on some level my whole life, but dad has taught me to take control of my life and to have hope. This year, the dedication and hard work of many research scientists validated my hope with the release of a new medication that has cured me of my migraines. Remember, for all that we as individuals with the help of our doctors can do now to help us live our best aging years, there will be even more strategies available tomorrow!

One of my senior patients said, "Mostly, I feel like an older teenager inside—all the great parts of being a teenager but not all the angst." Aging is a privilege, and how we do it matters. Feel free to take control of your aging process and your life, enjoy each moment, and hold on to hope. I want you to age like my dad, like fine wine or like delicious, aged cheese, not like sour grapes or moldy, old cheese in the back of your refrigerator. Embrace the changes of aging as your trophies of life—the gray hair, the wrinkles, and so on. But always remember that you are in control of how you live your life. This book is full of ideas for you to ponder, discuss with your doctor and to try out. Pick one challenge to address at a time. Then start by taking one idea at a time, incorporating it into your life and see how a small change can affect your well-being. I want to see you conquer aging, not by trying to be younger but instead by being the happiest, freest, healthiest, and most independent version of yourself you can be. I want you to live your best aging life.

This book began with the story of Mae, who, at ninety-three, still had marathon shoes. What will your version of Mae be? How are you going to get there?

RESOURCES

The information in this book is comprised of years of study. To stay current on the latest medical discoveries and innovations, I read:

For Medical Professionals

The New England Journal of Medicine: www.nejm.org

New England Journal Watch, which alerts me to thousands of the most influential scientific studies that come out each year across all of the medical journals: www.jwatch.org

Up-to-date medical resource: www.uptodate.com

For a General Audience

General Medicinal Information

- CDC.gov
- Mayoclinic.org
- Clevelandclinic.org
- Medscape.com
- WebMD.com
- MDConsult.com
- Emedicine.com

Advance Directives Tools

- www.fivewishes.org
- www.theconversationproject.org
- www.prepareforyourcare.org
- med.stanford.edu/letter.html
- www.getyourshittogether.org
- www.GoWish.org

Disease Society Specific Information

- Alzheimer's Association—www.alz.org
- American Association of Clinical Endocrinology—www.aace.com
- The North American Menopause Society—www.menopause.org/for-women
- Urology Care Foundation—www.urologyhealth.org

Information Specific to Aging

- Health in Aging—www.healthinaging.org

INDEX

ABOUT THE AUTHOR

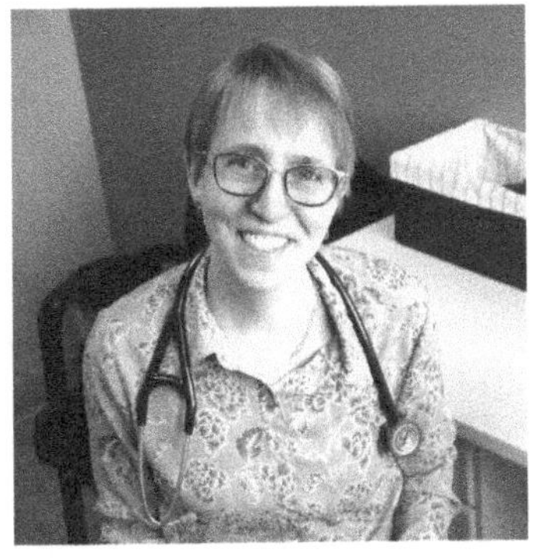

Jeannette Guerrasio, MD, is a primary care internal medicine physician in private practice in Denver, Colorado. She graduated from Albany Medical College and completed her residency at the University of Connecticut and a mini-geriatrics fellowship through the Reynolds Foundation at the University of California Los Angeles. While practicing at the University of Colorado, in the Department of Medicine, for thirteen years, she became a Professor of Medicine and was inducted into the Academy of Medical Educators. She is committed to the clinical care of patients, with expertise in both adult medicine and geriatrics, having done research to improve geriatric assessments and to decrease delirium, functional decline, and urinary tract infections.

Dr. Guerrasio is also an internationally known teacher and educator. She pioneered an approach to improve the educational experience of medical students and residents. She is the author of *Remediation of the Struggling Medical Learner*, editions 1 and 2, *Remediation Case Studies*, and countless book chapters and journal articles.

Visit her online at www.jeannetteguerrasiomd.com.